SURVIVING THE COVID PANDEMIC

Contents of a Diary

Third Edition

By Susan F Langlois

Published 2026

Contents

Glossary

211 – In Canada, a free, confidential helpline that connects people to vital government, health, and community services.

Age-friendly Orillia – An advisory committee of the Orillia City Council that considers both the challenges and opportunities of the city's aging population.

AIDS – Acquired Immunodeficiency Syndrome, the most advanced stage of infection caused by the Human Immunodeficiency Virus (HIV)

Airborne virus – infected respiratory particles that are suspended in the air. People can catch these viruses by simply inhaling them, even after the infected person leaves the area.

Alpha variant – A SARS-CoV-2 variant of Covid-19 virus.

Antigen – Any substance, such as a protein, sugar, or toxin, that is recognized by the immune system as foreign to the body.

BANAC – Barrie Area Native Advisory Circle, Ontario, is a regional indigenous health and social planning and implementation organization.

Care Plan – A documented, personalized guide outlining an individual's health needs, goals and interventions.

Carcinogenicity – The ability of an agent, substance or exposure to cause cancer or increase the risk of developing cancer.

CCAC – Continuing Care Access Centers is a single point of access for government-funded healthcare in Ontario.

CDC – Centers for Disease Control and Prevention is the leading national public health agency in the USA, designed to protect public health by preventing and controlling disease, injury or disability.

CERB – Canada Emergency Response Benefit was a temporary, federal relief program created by the Government of Canada to support employed and self-employed Canadians who lost their jobs or had their hours significantly reduced due to the COVID-19 pandemic.

COHT – Couchiching Ontario Health Team was introduced by the Ontario government in 2019, a model that intends to streamline and integrate the services of healthcare providers in the Ontario areas of Severn, Orillia, Rama First Nation, Ramara and Oro-Medonte.

COVID-19 – Coronavirus disease 2019, is a contagious respiratory illness caused by the coronavirus SARS-CoV-2. It was first detected in China in December 2019.

Delta variant – A variant of SARS-CoV-2 first detected in India in October 2020.

Emergent urgent surgery – Defines a newly appearing or suddenly occurring condition that requires time-critical urgent surgery to prevent a life-threatening situation or death.

Ethics – A philosophical study of moral principles that govern human behaviours, determining what is right, wrong, good or bad.

It provides the foundational framework used to navigate complex decisions, define our values, and evaluate our actions in daily life, society and professional fields.

FDA – Food and Drug Administration is a USA federal agency responsible for protecting public health by ensuring the safety, efficacy, and security of human and veterinary drugs, biological products, medical devices, the nation's food supply, cosmetics, and radiation-emitting products.

Gain of function – A scientific term describing a genetic alteration that gives an organism a new property or significantly enhances an existing one. The term is often used for research that makes a virus or microbe more transmissible, more virulent, able to infect a new host or better at evading immunity.

Gene Therapy – A medical technique that treats or cures diseases by altering a person's DNA. Instead of using drugs or surgery, it works by replacing, inactivating or introducing specific genes to stop the underlying cause of a condition at a cellular level. Gene therapy with RNA can modify gene expression to reduce harmful proteins or increase beneficial ones.

Health System Performance Network – A group funded by a grant from the Ontario Ministry of Health and Long-Term Care to assess policy directions and organizational strategies to guide efforts to improve health outcomes and patient experiences of care while containing costs.

HIV – Human Immunodeficiency Virus. Also refer to AIDS

Holistic - Addressing, treating, or considering the entire system or person rather than focusing solely on individual parts or symptoms. Often summarizing the idea "the whole is greater than the sum of its parts".

ICU – Intensive Care Unit of a hospital.

Integrated Health Care – A patient-focused, evidence-based approach that combines conventional medicine with safe, validated complementary therapies, such as acupuncture, yoga and meditation.

JAMA – Journal of the American Medical Association is a peer-reviewed medical journal, publishing biomedical research, reviews and editorials.

JET – Joint Executive Team, the lead group of the COHT. Also refer to COHT.

JUNO awards – Annual awards recognizing outstanding achievements in Canada's music industry.

Kapasi sarcoma – A type of cancer that forms in the cells lining blood vessels and lymph vessels, often showing up as red, purple or brown skin lesions or lesions in the mouth and internal organs.

LCBO – Liquor Control Board of Ontario is a Crown agency that retails and distributes alcoholic beverages throughout the Canadian province of Ontario.

LHIN – Local Health Integration Networks in Ontario are a regional health authority responsible for planning, funding and coordinating local health services. As of 2026, they have transitioned their planning functions to Ontario Health and now operate as Home and Community Care Support Services, focusing on home care delivery.

MAID – Medical Assistance in Dying is a legal end-of-life option in Canada that allows a person to receive medical help to end their life under specific conditions set out in the Criminal Code and Federal-provincial guidelines.

Metric – An adjective indicating relation to measurement in general, or a noun describing a specific type of measurement, as a measurement of the improvement in patient care.

Modernization Home and Community Care Act – The Ontario Government's plan to connect people in Ontario to the health care they need, when they need it.

mRNA – messenger RNA. It is the molecule that carries instructions from DNA to the cell's protein-making machinery, where those instructions are used to build proteins. Synthetic mRNA is also the basis of mRNA vaccines, which give cells instructions to make a piece of a virus.

N95 mask – A tight-fitting respirator that filters at least 95% of airborne particles, including very small particles greater than 0.3 microns (some viruses) when correctly fitted. It is designed to form a seal around the nose and mouth, so air goes through the filter instead of leaking around the edges. "N" means it is not resistant to oil. "95" means it filters at least 95% of test particles under standard conditions.

Negative pressure chamber – An isolation environment or room designed to keep contaminated air contained within a space by maintaining lower air pressure inside compared to the outside area. These chambers are used in hospitals for infectious disease control.

NIAID – National Institute of Allergy and Infectious Disease, is an agency in the USA that pursues the understanding, treating, and preventing infectious and immunologic diseases. It uses scientific approaches to address the causes of these diseases and ways to prevent, diagnose and treat them.

NIH – National Institutes of Health is the primary medical and biomedical research agency of the United States federal government. It is the largest public funder of biomedical research in the world.

OHT – Ontario Health Team. Also refer to COHT.

Ontario Crisis List – A top-priority, expedited waitlist for long-term care homes in Ontario for individuals requiring immediate admission due to significant safety risks. It is reserved for those whose care needs can no longer be met at home or who are facing an urgent discharge from a hospital.

Pandemic – An infectious disease outbreak that rapidly spreads across multiple countries or continents, affecting many people. It is essentially a global-scale epidemic (a large outbreak where a disease spreads rapidly to many people across a region or country).

Patient-centred care – A health care approach that prioritizes an individual's specific needs, values and preferences, making them the active partner in their own health decisions.

Patient Declaration of Values – A document, mandated by the province of Ontario, that outlines what patients, families and caregivers can expect from their healthcare experience, focusing on dignity, partnership, and high-quality care.

PCR test – A polymerase chain reaction test is a highly sensitive lab method used to detect genetic material (DNA or RNA) from pathogens, such as viruses or bacteria, in a sample. PCR amplifies tiny amounts of genetic material so they can be detected, even when only a very small number of viral particles are present.

PFAC – Patient and Family Advisory Committee

Plasmid DNA – A small, circular, double-stranded DNA molecule that exists separately from the main chromosome in cells, mostly commonly in bacteria. It can replicate autonomously and often carries genes that give the host cell a selective advantage, such as antibiotic-resistance or toxin-producing genes.

PM – Prime Minister

PSW – Personal Support Worker in Ontario is a frontline healthcare professional who provides essential daily care to individuals with illnesses, injuries or age-related needs, typically working in home care, long-term care or hospitals.

PVCC – Provincial Vaccine Contact Center in Ontario during the COVID-19 pandemic.

Palliative Care – Specialized medical care for people with a serious illness, focused on relieving symptoms, stress, and improving quality of life for both the patient and their family. It can be given at any stage of illness and alongside other treatments, not only at the end of life.

Quality – A job in quality control, quality assurance or inspection.

RAMA – The Chippewas of RAMA First Nation are an Indigenous community on the East Shore of Lake Simcoe in Ontario, Canada.

Regulatory Affairs – A profession and corporate department that ensures organizations comply with local and global legislative guidelines. Regulatory professionals act as the crucial bridge between scientific innovation and government authorities to safeguard public health. Regulatory affairs professionals are responsible for the entire lifecycle of a product.

Without regulatory affairs, safe and effective products would never successfully reach patients and consumers. They translate raw laboratory and clinical data into the exact legal and scientific language that government regulators need to trust and approve a product for public use. Professionals in this area constantly track evolving laws to protect the public from hazardous practices while ensuring companies can safely market their products.

Respiratory virus – The most common and frequent infections in humans. Hundreds of different viruses can be considered respiratory. The viruses enter through the respiratory tract. Measles and SARS ares examples of respiratory viruses.

Responsible Person – A key, legally designated figure responsible for ensuring that medicinal products are manufactured, tested, stored, transported, and distributed in compliance with applicable regulations and Good Manufacturing Practices. Ensuring compliance with national legislation and regulations of the importing countries. Deciding on the final disposition of returned, rejected or recalled products. Ensures safety, quality and potency of manufactured and released products.

RNA – Ribonucleic Acid is a molecule found in living cells that helps carry and use genetic information, especially in making proteins.

Roadmap to Reopen – A three-step plan during the COVID-19 pandemic that guided a safe and gradual reopening of the province of Ontario and lifting public health measures based on the province wide COVID-19 vaccination rate and improvements in key public health and health system indicators.

SARS – Severe Acute Respiratory Syndrome, a viral respiratory illness caused by a coronavirus.

SDH – Social Determinants of Health are the non-medical, social and economic factors that influence individual and community health outcomes. The key factors include income levels, housing stability, employment status, education, access to nutritious food and structural discrimination. These conditions profoundly shape a person's quality of life and health risks.

Science Table – A grid of rows and columns used to organize

numerical data or experimental results.

Snowbirds – A person who lives in a colder, northern part of North America and then moves to a warmer southern climate for the winter months and then returns home in the spring.

Spike Protein – A protein that sticks out from the surface of certain enveloped viruses forming club- or spike-like structures you see in illustrations of viruses like coronaviruses and influenza.

Synthetic RNA – An artificially created RNA produced in the lab rather than transcribed naturally inside cells.

Triage – A process of quickly assessing and prioritizing patients (or problems) based on the urgency of their need for care and likelihood of survival, so that limited resources are allocated to maximize the number of survivors.

Transitional Care – Care that bridges the gap between acute hospital stays and returning home or moving to long-term care, offering short-term, 24/7 support for medically stable patients who no longer need intense hospital services.

Vaccine – Traditional vaccines give the body the germ itself in a weakened or inactivated form, or just parts of it to trigger immunity to the virus, bacteria or microbe. mRNA vaccines work by giving the cells instructions to make a piece of the germ, usually a protein, so the immune system can learn to recognize it. Both types of vaccines are meant to train the immune system to respond faster if an infection is later encountered.

Ventilator – A machine that helps a person breathe, or breathes for them entirely, by moving air into and out of the lungs. A ventilator uses pressure to push air into the lungs.

VON – Victorian Order of Nurses is a Canadian non-profit organization that provides specialized home care, personal support, and community services. Operating mainly in Ontario and Nova Scotia, VON offers care to seniors, families and individuals, including nursing, Meals on Wheels and adult day programs.

Wet market – A market that sells fresh perishable foods like meat, fish, fruit, and vegetables and sometimes live animals. The term wet usually refers to water, ice and cleaning that keep those foods fresh and can leave the floors wet.

WHO – World Health Organization is the United Nations specialized agency responsible for international public health.

WWI – World War One was the deadliest and most destructive global conflict in history up to that time.

WWII – World War Two was the largest and deadliest war in history, with fighting across Europe, Africa, Asia and the Pacific.

Prologue

The devastation caused by the COVID-19 pandemic was over seven years in the making. Some said it was an unfortunate natural disaster, others claimed it was an experiment of global control, some blamed greed, and others spoke of a planned genocide. No matter which camp you are in, you likely agree that all those scenarios played their part. There were too many involved in the deceit, ignorance and naivety to blame any one person or persons, organization, government or country. That is what made the global COVID-19 pandemic the perfect storm.

One evening in March 2020, while binge-watching one of our favourite comedy series and checking the news on our tablets, I turned to my husband and said that I needed to start a daily diary. He asked me why a diary. I said I had a feeling that this new virus reported in China may become a problem of global importance. Little did I know that the event would change the world in so many negative ways and exceed the damage of both WWI and WWII, combined.

At the beginning of the COVID-19 pandemic, I put my trust in the government, regulatory professionals, the medical community and popular news outlets. They wooed us with partial truths and appeared to be following the standard practices when rolling out a new vaccine.

Slow and steady; beginning to vaccinate seniors and those with other health issues that may put them at risk of severe disease, not recommending it for pregnant women, children, those with autoimmune disorders, compromised immune systems or allergies. Then they made the vaccine available for anyone who wanted it once the front-line health care workers, long-term care workers and long-term care residents were offered it.

I slowly realized that nothing they told us was as it seemed. They lied by omission, and I initially fell for their lies. Once I realized this, I began to question everything. It was a very slow awakening for me, but once the journey commenced, it rapidly accelerated.

When the US and Canadian governments first announced in February 2020 that a new COVID-19 "vaccine" would be released within the next ten months, my Spidey sense was activated. Then, in early December 2020, I learned that the first two of the vaccines on offer were produced using a synthetic messenger RNA platform.

When the release announcement was made, I discovered that in 2013, the FDA established that the regulation of gene therapy products did not apply to "vaccines" against infectious diseases. This established a precedent that enabled the mRNA -19 spike protein to be classified as a vaccine – rather than a traditional

gene therapy product – thereby exempting it from several safety and effectiveness regulations.

Gene therapy changes cells to treat a disease. A vaccine trains the immune system to prevent a disease.

An mRNA vaccine trains cells to produce the spike protein that, in turn, trains the immune system.

A traditional vaccine uses a spike protein or antigen to directly train the immune system.

A gene therapy product is generally reviewed under gene-therapy-specific rules with extra focus on genetic risk, including:

carcinogenicity,

persistence of effect,

tissue distribution, and

long-term patient follow-up.

A vaccine is regulated as a short-term product with review centered on safety in healthy people and immune response rather than therapeutic effect. Regulators focus more on whether the product induces protection against a disease.

Another major difference is the dose of spike protein or antigen.

One dose of a vaccine contains the same amount of antigen every

time, and the regulators test for consistency and potency of each dose. Each person responds to that antigen differently depending on their previous exposure to the antigen and the state of their immune system.

In the case of an mRNA vaccine, the body's cells become the manufacturing plant producing the spike protein or antigen, and there is no control for dose consistency from person to person. Each person responds to the spike protein differently, depending on their previous exposure to the spike protein and the state of their immune system. Some may not make spike protein, and others may make too much of it.

To add insult to injury, regulators created an Emergency Release regulation which allowed many shortcuts and exempted the "vaccine" from informed consent, product recall and liability.

The government also introduced mandates and coercion.

Prior to the Covid pandemic, no mRNA vaccine had been approved due to safety and effectiveness issues.

The pandemic provided an opportunity to fast-track this new technology and to establish a foothold on the market. My concern increased as I realized that once the mRNA Covid vaccine was introduced on the market, no additional safety data would be required to obtain regulatory approval for other

vaccines made using the same technology.

My loss of trust inspired me to continue documenting the events in a diary, which takes the reader through a fascinating and troubling journey.

The Epilogue at the end of this transcription summarizes the important take-away components of the Covid pandemic and may be one of the most important Chapters in this book.

About The Author

Before delving into the contents of this book, the reader should understand a bit about me and why my family and friends encouraged me to publish my experience during the COVID-19 pandemic.

My name is Susan Langlois, and I grew up in Toronto, Ontario, Canada. I spent my adult life working in the city I called home, retired from my forty-five-year career in 2017 and moved to Orillia, Ontario, Canada.

My career in the biotech industry concentrated on managing quality control, global clinical trials and international regulatory approvals.

I spent the first twenty years in a Canadian company, Connaught Laboratories Limited, that manufactured and distributed vaccines and immunotherapeutic products around the world.

I worked closely with:

Canadian and USA regulatory agencies,

EU regulators,

the World Health Organization,

Ministries of Health,

health insurance companies,

health care institutions,

and hundreds of physicians.

By the time I left Connaught in 1992, I was accountable for the release of every batch of product produced by the company and held the position of Director Regulatory Affairs and Responsible Person.

I became one of the most knowledgeable biologics regulatory professionals in North America before the age of forty.

To add to my experience, I obtained –

an Executive Business Certificate from the University of Western Ontario, and

A Regulatory Affairs Professional Certificate from the US Regulatory Affairs Professional Society.

Prior to beginning my career, I obtained:

A Laboratory Technologist certificate from Humber College, and

A Basic Immunology certificate from the Toronto Institute of Medical Technology.

When I left Connaught to become a biotech consultant, I was immediately offered a Vice President position in a start-up company. My role was to manage the regulatory, quality and clinical operations of a synthesized red blood cell substitute. I accepted the position and continued working with them for six years.

My next adventure was as Vice President of a medical device company developing an immunotherapy. My role was to manage regulatory, clinical trials and quality. This position honed my ability to navigate combination products and immune therapies through their complex regulatory pathways. I spent ten years with this company.

After thirty-six years in the biotech industry, I decided to try something different.

I joined a research foundation and managed the selection and oversight of promising projects for prostate cancer. I spent six years in this role, where I learned much about cancer and its related research and industries.

I concluded my career by holding a few contract positions in the biotech industry, which allowed me to update my regulatory and clinical trial knowledge.

Prior to my retirement, I was an advocate for both my dad and my husband's father during their final stages of prostate cancer and palliative care prior to their death.

After my retirement, I was a caregiver to my mother, who suffered from mobility issues and early-onset dementia. When she reached her ninetieth birthday, I moved her from the home I was raised in to an assisted living facility and then to a palliative care facility before she passed in May 2021.

In 2017, when I decided to retire, my husband and I moved to Orillia, Ontario, Canada. My plan was to give back to the community that supported my career, and I spent the next six years:

As a volunteer porter at our local hospital,

Working with patients in various hospital areas, including the emergency, diagnostic, renal dialysis, cancer care, pediatric and geriatric departments,

As a member of the hospital Ethics Committee, Operations Committee, and Patient Advisory Committee,

Working with the Couchiching Ontario Health Team, and as an advisor to the Ontario Ministry of Health.

During the pandemic, I was an advisor for the local Couchiching Ontario Health Team's

Community outreach and engagement programs,

Covid testing,

Covid vaccination,

Triage processes,

Hospital operations,

Hospital outpatient and visitor policy development.

After 2017, I received no compensation for my services, which allowed unrestricted actions that often resulted in negative outcomes.

Chapter 1

MY DIARY

During December 2019, my son's family visited us in Orillia over the Christmas holidays. They were all recovering from a bad case of the flu, so I jokingly said that maybe they visited a wet market and caught the Chinese virus. A few weeks later, this joke was considered in extremely poor taste.

In early January 2020, life was unaffected by the Chinese virus.

I was appointed Volunteer Chair of the Patient and Caregiver Advisory Committee for the Couchiching Ontario Health Team and needed to add members to the committee. In that role, I conducted interviews with patients and patient caregivers in our community.

During the interviews, many of the individuals provided suggestions for the Health Team. There were many areas of concern, including:

communication,

transparency,

reliability,

emergency wait times,

ethics framework,

MAID,

palliative care,

home visits for seniors,

home care,

access to specialists and family physicians,

access to medical records,

navigating the system,

wait times for long-term care,

and quality of care.

In other words, the Ontario Health Care system was collapsing.

On January 23, the first case of COVID-19 in Canada was admitted to Sunnybrook Hospital in Toronto and placed into a negative pressure chamber. The patient was a fifty-year-old male who had recently returned from Wuhan, China. He was admitted to the Emergency Department after a rapid onset of symptoms.

It was confirmed on January 27 by the Public Health Agency of Canada's National Microbiology Laboratory in Winnipeg, using a PCR test, that he had COVID-19.

The man's wife was also infected. On January 31, the third and fourth cases in Canada were reported.

On January 30, WHO declared a global health emergency.

There were frequent mentions in the news about a very contagious and deadly virus that originated in China. It was claimed that the virus originated in a wet market. That claim was followed by suspicion that the virus was manmade and leaked from a research lab in Wuhan.

The World Health Organization was monitoring the situation and claimed that the virus most probably originated from the wet market. The National Institutes of Health in the US denied the likelihood that the virus was manmade and came from a lab they used in Wuhan, China. The numerous denials strengthened the suspicions that the US scientists working on COVID-19 gain-of-function experiments in the Wuhan lab accidentally or intentionally leaked the virus.

These suspicions were further supported by US President Trump, who downplayed the seriousness of the virus. He blamed China and claimed that there was a cover-up by the Chinese government.

On February 7, a plane carrying more than two hundred Canadians from Wuhan arrived in Trenton, Ontario, and they were quarantined for fourteen days. On February 20, a woman who returned from Iran became the sixth case of COVID-19 and the first person in Canada who did not recently visit China or come in contact with someone who did.

I sensed this virus was unusual and felt compelled to track its development. One night in March 2020, I told my husband that I would start a daily diary to record the number of cases and deaths worldwide. I planned to keep the diary for a few months, until the daily number of cases dropped.

By March 8, there were several cases in people who did not go to China or come in contact with someone who did. On that date, the first death in Canada from COVID-19 was reported. The man in his eighties died in a nursing home.

When the US and Canadian governments first announced in February 2020 that a new COVID-19 "vaccine" would be released within the next ten months, my Spidey sense was activated. Then, in early December 2020, I learned that the first two of the vaccines on offer were produced using a synthetic messenger RNA platform.

When the release announcement was made, I discovered that in 2013, the FDA established that the regulation of gene therapy products did not apply to “vaccines” against infectious diseases. This established a precedent that enabled the mRNA COVID-19 spike protein to be classified as a vaccine – rather than a traditional gene therapy product – thereby exempting it from several safety and effectiveness regulations.

Gene therapy changes cells to treat a disease. A vaccine trains the immune system to prevent a disease.

An mRNA vaccine trains cells to produce the spike protein that, in turn, trains the immune system.

A traditional vaccine uses a spike protein or antigen to directly train the immune system.

A gene therapy product is generally reviewed under gene-therapy specific rules with extra focus on genetic risk, including:

carcinogenicity,

persistence of effect,

tissue distribution, and

long-term patient follow-up.

A vaccine is regulated as a short-term product with review centered on safety in healthy people and immune response rather than therapeutic effect. Regulators focus more on whether the product induces protection against a disease.

Another major difference is the dose of spike protein or antigen.

One dose of a vaccine contains the same amount of antigen every time, and the regulators test for consistency and potency of each dose. Each person responds to that antigen differently depending on their previous exposure to the antigen and the state of their immune system.

In the case of an mRNA vaccine, the body's cells become the

manufacturing plant producing spike protein or antigen, and there is no control for dose consistency from person to person. Each person responds to the spike protein differently, depending on their previous exposure to the spike protein and the state of their immune system. Some may not make spike protein, and others may make too much of it.

To add insult to injury, regulators created an “Emergency Release” regulation which allowed many shortcuts and exempted the "vaccine" from informed consent, product recall and liability.

The government also introduced mandates and coercion.

Prior to the COVID-19 pandemic, no mRNA vaccine had been approved due to safety and effectiveness concerns.

The pandemic provided an opportunity to fast-track this new technology and to establish a foothold in the market. My apprehension increased as I realized that once the mRNA COVID-19 vaccine was introduced on the market, no additional safety data would be required to obtain regulatory approval for other vaccines made using the same technology.

As the pandemic persisted, I participated in

several health care committees,

advocating for seniors,

communicating concerns about the handling of the pandemic and vaccines,

navigating my mom's decline and eventual death, and

reporting health news on a call-in Seniors News Line.

My loss of trust inspired me to continue documenting the daily events in a diary.

In the remaining chapters of this book, the events are presented in the order and as written in my personal log. At the beginning, most of my entries were simply a record of the management of the pandemic.

As 2020 progressed, the entries became more detailed, and my frustration more apparent.

The Epilogue at the end of this transcription summarizes the important take-away components of the COVID-19 pandemic, and combined with the Prologue, may be one of the most important Chapters in this book.

I did not attempt to verify any of the notes recorded in my daily diary. All opinions, when expressed, are my own.

I did not develop a Bibliography of supporting references for this book, because all the information contained herein was obtained from personal experience, public announcements or my own opinions.

There is a Glossary at the beginning of the book which provides an alphabetical list of most of the acronyms and technical jargon mentioned in the text.

I make no representations or warranties, either express or implied, with respect to the accuracy, completeness, currency, reliability or usefulness of the information contained in this book.

Chapter 2

MARCH 2020

March 11

The World Health Organization declared the novel COVID-19 a pandemic.

March 12

Canadian Prime Minister Trudeau announced that he is undertaking self-isolation measures following his wife's positive COVID-19 test upon her return from England. Most sports leagues suspended their season, and the JUNO awards were cancelled. The Ontario government announced that schools are closed across the province for two weeks after the March school break.

March 13

The Canadian Federal government announced that Parliament will take a break and urged Canadians currently abroad to return home as soon as possible.

March 15

The province of Nova Scotia, Canada, reported its first three cases.

March 16

All public spaces in Ontario, Canada, are ordered closed, hospitals have cancelled all elective surgeries and diagnostic procedures, and the Canadian border is closed to non-Canadians.

March 17

I joined a hospital laboratory discussion about the blood shortage caused by the postponement of donations.

Both provinces, Ontario and Alberta, have declared states of emergency.

I sense that the COVID-19 pandemic will be remembered as a major international event in modern times.

March 18

Canada and the US closed their shared border to all non-essential traffic.

March 19

Provinces, Ontario and New Brunswick declared a State of Emergency, as did our local Simcoe County. Everyone was ordered to stay in their homes except for essential services.

March 20

COVID-19 cases passed one thousand across the country.

The province of Manitoba declared a state of emergency.

Hospitals introduced strict access rules effective today. Visitors are no longer permitted to enter the hospital. Patients, including those who are dying, may only speak to their family by phone or tablet.

All volunteers, including me, were ordered to stay home. They will not call us back until after the crisis is over.

March 21

The town of Orillia, where I live, declared a State of Emergency.

The Orillia Soldiers Memorial Hospital, our local hospital, announced that a COVID-19 assessment center will be open in two days.

Everything is shut down, and all citizens are ordered to remain home for fourteen days UNLESS essential needs are required.

I called a local city councillor about setting up a daily telephone call-in news program for seniors and those who do not have access to the internet or cable. Local newspapers are closed, so this would keep the vulnerable updated.

March 22

A neighbour provided a list of contact information for our neighbourhood. I emailed them a coronavirus update and told them that I would send them new information as it becomes available. Side note - I sat on the Ontario Health Care Team and attended the Hospital Staff meetings, so I was privy to information that was not in the news.

The Ministry of Health reported that social distancing will probably not end for months. Two cases were reported in Orillia. The news reported that Snowbirds, Canadians who live in the state of Florida during the winter months, are returning to Canada potentially infected with COVID-19.

March 23

I went to the hospital for an ultrasound. It was very eerie with empty hallways, and the few I did see were in full protective gear. I underwent a COVID-19 screening through a series of questions and was instructed to wear a disposable surgical mask prior to being granted entry.

Ottawa announced repatriation flights for Canadians stranded in foreign countries.

March 24

Today, there were over 400,000 cases and over 19,000 deaths reported worldwide. Italy, the USA, Germany and France have reported the greatest number of cases and deaths.

Both Federal and Provincial governments are closing all non-essential businesses, and they are offering financial initiatives, including postponement of taxes, mortgage, hydro and water payments.

The Olympics are officially postponed until 2021.

India has locked down their entire country for twenty-one days.

I spoke to a city councillor on the phone again about the start of the telephone news line for seniors. I volunteered to provide daily health updates for those without access to the internet.

Several new cases were reported in Ontario, and the number rose from eighty-five to one hundred in twenty-four hours.

March 25

Canada made it mandatory for all travellers arriving in Canada to quarantine for fourteen days.

March 26

I am preparing for an Operations Committee meeting by video conference. It is essential to examine the frameworks adopted by other hospitals during the pandemic, particularly regarding criteria for allocating treatments or beds when resources are scarce.

March 30

Over the weekend, COVID-19 reached 150,000 cases in the US and over 7,000 in Canada. Ontario has over 1,700 cases. Orillia had four deaths, two of whom worked with me as volunteers at the hospital and had many pre-existing health issues.

I am reviewing triage protocols for the hospital Ethics Committee.

The province now controls authority previously held by the hospitals. The March 28 protocol is intricate and troubling and forces decisions about who will receive treatment based on perceived value to society, age and other co-existing health issues.

PM Trudeau said that a new wage subsidy program will cover all businesses whose revenue has dropped more than thirty percent because of COVID-19.

March 31

Nineteen deaths occurred in the town of Bobcaygeon's long-term care facility.

My mom's assisted-living retirement home suggested that those who want to take their family member home should do so immediately before a case occurs there. However, there is a catch. Once they leave, they will not be allowed to return. We decided it was best for Mom to remain in quarantine where she is.

Chapter 3

APRIL 2020

April 1

COVID-19 case numbers in the US have increased significantly, reaching over 200,000 cases and over 4,000 deaths. Canada has reached close to 10,000 cases and over 50 deaths. China's situation has not changed, and some speculate that information about the number of cases may be withheld.

April 2

Trump publicly admitted that he is afraid of the COVID-19 virus and that he is accepting advice from a panel of experts.

The global number of cases has reached one million today with over 50,000 deaths.

April 3

I attended a hospital Operations Committee meeting today by video conference and these were the highlights:

No nonmedical staff will be assigned to cases.

We need a group of Ethics Committee members available 24/7.

We will follow provincial PPE guidelines and not exceed them.

No reprocessing or sterilizing of N95 masks will be performed.

Re-use of masks by the same person will be allowed.

I expressed my concern about the validity of reprocessing or re-using N95 masks, explaining that there are no data to support either scenario. The staff pointed out that they have no choice. Until the government provides adequate supplies of Personal Protection Equipment (PPE), they will re-use the N95 masks. I added that this poses a high infection risk to staff, something that I am certain they did not need to hear.

In the afternoon, first responders held a parade of emergency vehicles around Orillia Soldiers Memorial Hospital to demonstrate their appreciation of staff caring for COVID-19 patients. Hospital staff watched from the windows, and the President of the hospital later stated that the support was heartwarming. Similar demonstrations of support occurred all over the country because nurses and doctors were considered heroes.

By bedtime, the US reported 278,000 cases and 7,400 deaths, and Canada reported 12,500 cases and 208 deaths.

Ontario Premier Ford announced that there will be more closures by midnight tomorrow.

April 4

Yesterday, President Trump ordered 3M, the US-based science and manufacturing company, to keep all N95 masks in the US and to stop all deliveries to Canada.

PM Trudeau signed a contract with Amazon to deliver all PPE supplies needed in Canada.

April 5

The number of cases continues to climb, and more areas are closed today in Orillia, including the Orillia public marina and boat launches until May 31.

Pharmacies are limiting drug refills to thirty days due to shortages caused by shutdowns.

April 6

3M made a deal with Trump to continue providing N95 masks to Canada.

It was reported that the Prime Minister of England is in the Intensive Care Unit (ICU) due to Covid-19 and Prince Charles of England has recovered from COVID-19.

April 7

Currently, there have been approximately 1,500,000 reported cases and more than 80,000 fatalities worldwide.

April 8

There is an Ethics Committee Triage Team meeting today by video conference. We discussed several COVID-19 cases needing a ventilator. There are insufficient ventilators available, so we applied the triage framework provided by the province, and the process proved to be challenging. I would prefer not to be responsible for informing patients that they did not satisfy the selection criteria.

Many individuals are now making cloth masks to assist in mitigating the transmission of illness by asymptomatic persons, and the government and health authorities are encouraging this. Homemade cloth masks do not prevent virus transmission and may encourage unsafe socializing by providing false comfort.

Virus-sized particles are typically less than 0.1 micron in size.

Cloth masks, depending on the fabric, block only 50 to 70% of large droplets (greater than 20 microns) from coughs or sneezes. In addition, cloth masks can harbour moisture-trapped virus, risking contamination upon removal.

Surgical masks perform slightly better than cloth but leave gaps around the nose and mouth.

N95 masks (or respirators) perform the best. If they are fitted properly, they hug tightly around the nose and mouth and use electrostatic filtration.

April 9

Canada has started an Immunoglobulin clinical trial using a

recovered COVID-19 patient's plasma for severe cases. There is no information provided about when we will know the results. Side note – the results of the trial conducted by Sunnybrook Health Sciences in Toronto were inconclusive.

Ottawa projected that 4,400 to 44,000 Canadians could die of COVID-19. These unsupported predictions were meant to put fear into people's minds, making it easier to ensure compliance with government orders. They also announced that more than one million people lost their jobs in March 2020.

April 11

President Trump declared a State of Emergency for all fifty states. There have been 20,000 deaths nationwide, an increase from 10,000 in just five days.

April 12

Nurses worldwide have shared videos of themselves dancing in hospital hallways to show resilience. While these videos gained attention, many on social media criticized them for seeming joyful during times of patient deaths, highlighting how swiftly public opinion can shift.

April 13

The Canadian federal government announced that nearly 5.4 million Canadians will receive Canada Emergency Response Benefits

(CERB).

April 15

Canada passed one thousand COVID-19 deaths.

April 16

I joined a video conference with the Couchiching Ontario Health Team, COHT.

I suggested they establish a separate facility to perform diagnostics and uncomplicated procedures not requiring a general anesthetic. This would reduce the burden on hospital staff and allow more capacity for surgeries and critical care. The suggestion was rejected because if they move procedures outside the hospital, they will receive less money from the government. I was disappointed that money was considered a higher priority than patient care.

We discussed the vulnerable population in retirement and long-term care (LTC) homes. They require the most protection during the pandemic.

Soldiers Memorial Hospital is concerned about the summer months. The local Simcoe, Ontario, area population typically increases by an additional five thousand during the summer months. The hospital staff fears that people who own property north of Orillia will go to their cottages and stop in Orillia to shop. This will further increase the risk of more visits to the emergency department or new COVID-

19 cases.

The good news is that boating is closed, and hotels are not accepting leisure reservations; only corporate and essential workers are accepted.

Virtual assessments will be required for LTC patients before they are sent to the Emergency department.

April 20

Nineteen people were killed in mass shootings on Sunday night in the Canadian province of Nova Scotia. This incident is just one indication that mental health has deteriorated since the pandemic began.

April 22

Ontario and Quebec requested military assistance for LTC homes during the pandemic.

The number of cases reported globally has exceeded 2.6 million, and the number of total deaths has exceeded 180,000.

The Canadian federal government has declared it will invest one billion dollars in vaccine testing. I'm curious to know which companies will benefit from this funding.

April 25

I am having fun watching the white house staff 'moonwalk' back from Trump's recent comments that there should be studies to determine if injection of disinfectants into the body or applying heat and "powerful" UV light could cure COVID-19.

April 27

I made a delivery to my mom and had to leave it outside by the front door of the retirement home. In the parking lot, I chatted with staff and a transport provider for people with mobility challenges. He was waiting to take a client for a hospital x-ray and shared unsettling stories of anxious faces looking out from retirement and LTC home windows.

April 28

Canada reaches 50,000 cases.

One of our city councillors called and asked me to test the new Senior News phone number, and we discussed the launch and promotion of the program.

April 30

I attended the hospital Patient and Family Advisory Committee meeting via video conference, where patients raised concerns that echoed issues about the new mask and visitor policies I had previously mentioned at the Operations meeting.

Trump announced today that he is "in charge of fast-tracking" Covid-19 vaccines.

Chapter 4

MAY 2020

May 1

I participated in the hospital Operations Committee via video.

Emergent urgent surgeries, which handle immediate life-threats like trauma or conditions needing surgery within a narrow timeframe, are still ongoing.

Orilla may now re-establish elective surgery and diagnostics procedures due to the low COVID-19 incidence rate. However, without the availability of testing for COVID-19 and adequate PPE supplies, things will need to remain status quo.

Cancer Care Ontario is assessing patients individually to determine who needs care most and which procedures will be most effective.

The hospital will decide which procedures to bring back.

Approval from the province depends on the availability of resources.

The hospital may also need to support seniors in homes and other regions.

The hospital must set criteria for permitted procedures once approval is given.

May 2

Ontario marinas were given the ok to open on May 4.

The Ontario plans for hospitals to increase services are contingent on a continued decrease in new cases over the next fourteen days, adequate PPE supplies and availability of COVID-19 testing.

May 4

The restrictions were lifted in several but not all provinces.

May 5

The number of cases and deaths is still rising in Ontario.

May 6

Cottagers in Ontario are starting to head north from the big cities. Marinas are preparing to open, but are not allowed to let the public access their boats and island cottagers are denied access.

I called the dentist to schedule a repair for my broken front tooth, but there was no answer, so I emailed them instead.

May 8

Canada's unemployment rate is 13%, the second highest on record.

May 9

My dentist replied to my email, explained that the practice has been closed until safety protocols are in place, and scheduled my tooth repair for next week.

May 10

Tom's youngest sister informed us that their brother was hospitalized and tested for COVID-19. We have no further details and are quite concerned.

May 11

I called the wife of Tom's brother. His brother is now home in bed and under quarantine. He called us later, and we spoke for quite a while. He was not given any results from the COVID-19 test and was just told to quarantine himself.

May 12

The US has reached 80,000 deaths. Canada is nearing 5,000 deaths.

I am participating in an Ethics Committee Triage meeting by video this afternoon. I hate these meetings.

May 13

Ontario health officials have linked an inflammatory vasculitis in children who are positive for COVID-19.

Canada's top doctor says Canadians in areas where COVID-19 is still spreading should wear non-surgical, cloth masks at all times.

During a meeting with the hospital staff, I challenged the use of non-surgical masks and was told that, due to the PPE supply issues in hospitals and for first responders, they do not want the public to use them. They realize that the cloth masks do not work well, but they will at least help to control the panic. I checked the source of surgical masks and discovered that they all come from China. Is that just a coincidence, considering the virus came from China?

May 14

I went to the dentist. They had installed air filtration systems in every room and heavy plastic barriers across every entrance. They were all wearing PPE, including N95 masks. When I asked, I was told that they had their own source of N95 masks. Only one patient was allowed to enter the building at any one time. They locked the front door, and I had to call them to let them know I was in the parking lot. They buzzed me in when the last patient had vacated the building. There were very few employees inside. It was like entering a science fiction movie set. The dentist installed a temporary filling on my broken front tooth. We discussed a root canal that will have to wait until the COVID-19 risks are gone. At least the lisp is gone, and I sound more like myself again.

I spoke to Mom today. She is getting much worse. Her hallucinations are incredible and dark. Locked in her room with no visitors is causing a rapid decline in her condition. She was not hallucinating before the lockdowns. Prior to the lockdowns, I was visiting every day to provide stimulation and distraction. I was also monitoring her care. I wonder how much longer this will go on and worry about what impact the lockdown is having on her well-being.

May 15

Today, US President Trump announced the creation of Operation Warp Speed. He unveiled the public-private partnership aimed at accelerating the development, manufacture and distribution of COVID-19 vaccines with the goal of having them available by January 2021. All my experience does not allow me to imagine a vaccine that would be fully tested for safety and effectiveness in less than one year. Operation Warp Speed did not mention the testing. When challenged about the timeline, Dr. Fauci said that they would not take any shortcuts. He did not look comfortable when asked the question. I wonder why?

I participated in the Operations conference call regarding surgeries. We discussed my previous questions regarding patient safety, masks and visitors. A list of priority questions will be sent to the Ontario provincial Health Minister this weekend.

Surgeries may restart as early as Tuesday. I sent an email to the Ethics Committee providing a heads-up about the restart of surgeries, which may create many more ethical decisions for the team.

May 16

Many things are scheduled to reopen in Ontario this weekend, including parks, marinas, boating, elective surgeries, veterinary clinics, dog groomers and stores with curbside service.

May 18

Elisa Perego, a patient advocate in Italy, reported persistent symptoms following Covid-19 infection and complained that her condition was not recognized by the medical community. She was scorned and accused of spreading misinformation. She labelled the condition "Long-Covid" and created a support group on Twitter for anyone with the same symptoms. The group quickly grew to thousands.

May 19

Many stores reopened in Ontario.

May 21

The Couchiching Ontario Health Team meetings restarted today using video conference. We will discuss listening to patient voices and redesigning care.

May 22

The President of Orillia Soldiers Memorial Hospital sent me an article he drafted for my review and comments. He plans to submit it to the local news reporters. As requested, I added the work I am doing with the Patient Caregiver Advisory Committee of the Couchiching Ontario Health Team.

May 23

Thousands packed one of the largest parks in Toronto, creating fears of a new outbreak.

May 25

I took some food and pet toys to the local animal shelter. Unfortunately, there are many people surrendering their animals and very few making donations.

May 26

A new report from the Canadian military personnel helping LTC homes in Ontario revealed extreme neglect and exposed the extent of the horrific conditions facing residents.

I participated in the first “Surgery Start-up” meeting via video. We will meet daily until all the issues are resolved.

May 29

I reviewed the draft Patient Information Form for the COVID-19 vaccine and sent the Start-up team several comments related to COVID-19 screening and mask mandates.

One of my major concerns was about the instructions provided for intramuscular injection of the vaccine. When injecting a product that should remain in the muscle and not enter the bloodstream, as is the case for vaccines, the needle of the syringe containing the product should be inserted into the muscle. Before injection, the plunger should be pulled back to ensure that no blood is present. This would indicate that a vein had been entered. In that event, the needle should be removed, and the procedure should be repeated at a different site. Only when no blood is present should the product be injected. The manufacturer's instructions, as approved by the regulators, did not include this precaution. I asked the staff if the correct procedure was followed for the COVID-19 vaccine, and I was told that it would take too much time during mass vaccination. Although misplacement of intramuscular injections is rare when experienced staff is performing the procedure, injection of mRNA into the bloodstream is a major safety concern and may result in serious adverse events or long-term complications. I expressed my concern to the staff. Unfortunately, the injection procedure as described by the manufacturer would be the same wherever the vaccine is administered, and it will be impossible for me to communicate my concern to everyone. I was shocked that the regulators had not identified this as a concern.

May 31

I tried to renew our vehicle license plate stickers. The service department is closed, and the online site is not working.

Chapter 5

JUNE 2020

June 1

I donated more pet food to the animal shelter, and they were very grateful. Donations have been way down since the pandemic was announced, so they are encouraging people to donate money online.

June 4

I attended another video conference with the hospital Staff this afternoon. There is so much to be organized before non-urgent elective surgeries and major procedures can be restarted. The PPE supplies are still critical.

June 6

Mom's nurse called at 7:00 am. Mom fell in her room and was found on the floor. No one was there to witness the fall, so they will put her on "head watch". The residents are behind closed doors in their rooms, night and day, with very little monitoring. All their meals are brought to their rooms, and no one watches to see if they are eating or drinking.

June 11

I participated in a meeting with hospital operations staff today, and we discussed the progress of surgeries, triage, visitors and patient screening. During the meeting, I raised a concern that masks worn by staff may be a problem for children, patients who are deaf or patients with mental disorders or dementia. There was a suggestion that they look into clear plastic masks for these patients.

June 12

Ontario just entered stage two of its reopening, except for Toronto, Windsor and Peel.

June 17

New neighbours are moving in next door to our house. The elderly lady who previously lived there alone moved into my mom's retirement home last year. She had mobility issues but had all her mental faculties. She used to see one of her two daughters daily, but since the pandemic started, she has not had anyone visiting her. I wonder how she is doing now.

June 18

I had three conference calls today:

Hospital Operations,

Couchiching Ontario Health Team, and

Patient and Family Advisory Committee.

All the meetings were focused on the start-up of surgeries, visitor policies, and management of COVID-19 cases and assessments.

Canada has recorded more than 100,000 cases since the beginning of the pandemic.

June 22

The hospital will try out a new visitor procedure. Patients who have not seen their families since March 22 will be taken to the courtyard to meet with one member of their family. Distancing will be practiced, and the visit will be limited to thirty minutes. The strict criteria will limit the number of patients who may participate.

June 24

Mom's nurse called to tell me that Mom was acting like she may have had a transient ischemic attack (TIA). I asked them to take a urine sample and test for a urinary tract infection (UTI). In the elderly, the symptoms of a UTI may be the same as those of a TIA. It is disconcerting that I needed to ask for these tests.

June 26

The Canadian Red Cross sent 900 people to replace the military staff working in Quebec LTC homes until mid-September.

June 29

One of the hospital volunteers called to let me know that one of the other volunteers was found dead on his back deck. He lived alone; he did not go out or have any visitors since the pandemic started, and he had not been seen for a few days. I wondered how many others are in the same situation.

Chapter 6

JULY 2020

July 1

It is Canada Day, and we do not feel like celebrating.

I sent an email to the hospital President about masks. I pointed out that the cloth masks worn by patients are not adequate to prevent viruses from spreading. Disposable surgical masks may be a bit better at preventing spread. N95 masks fitted properly and worn for only a few hours prevent the spread. N95 masks, improperly fitted, reused or re-sterilized, may be worse than not wearing any mask at all. Masks also cause problems for people with dementia and hearing or breathing problems. Children's anxiety is worsened by masks worn by them and by the staff. The use of clear masks may help reduce some of these issues. Clear masks would allow the wearer to show their expression and make lip-reading possible. He committed to investigating my concerns.

July 2

I chatted with a former research colleague of mine about the COVID-19 virus and mask efficacy. I consider him an expert because he has a PhD in immunology and virology. He agreed with my concerns.

I participated in the Hospital Operations meeting and raised my concerns about masks in the hospital and how it effects patient care. My concerns landed on deaf ears. They are just following Ontario provincial orders.

July 4

After dinner, my husband and I took a ride to see the Orillia Port and Lakefront Park. The boat slips were empty, the park was very busy, and the downtown area was like a ghost town. Everything was closed.

July 9

I participated in the Hospital Operations video call. My issues about the masks were not discussed. I am starting to wonder what my role on the committee really is. Is my presence just symbolic?

We received our parking permit in the mail. All residents of Orillia must display the permit to be allowed to park free in the city. The town council is attempting to discourage visitors from the Toronto area by charging them a high parking fee.

July 15

I called the supervisor of the hospital volunteers to ask when we could get back to work. She said that they are considering ending the volunteer program indefinitely. The staff has been managing since the beginning of the year, and management does not think that the return of volunteers will be necessary. I wonder if the staff agree. We volunteer reduced the staff's workload significantly in the past. Since the pandemic started, they have had more responsibility and restrictions with fewer staff. It is probably just a liability issue because we are not paid employees, and we are not covered by their insurance.

July 16

Prime Minister Trudeau announced that the federal and provincial governments reached a deal to contribute billions of dollars in transfers to reopen the economy.

July 18

The Province of Quebec mandated mask-wearing in all indoor public places.

The Toronto Blue Jays baseball team was denied approval to play in Toronto due to the pandemic.

July 20

I drafted recommendations for Joint Executive Team (JET) consideration and approval. The gist of the document was to restart the Couchiching Ontario Health Team (COHT) Patient Family Advisory Committee (PFAC) now that the lockdowns have ended. I am currently the only member. As we restart elective surgeries and procedures, it is more important than ever that we obtain feedback and input from patients and caregivers. We also need to obtain feedback about the procedures and policies introduced during the pandemic.

I received the first invoice from the nurse I hired to cut Mom's nails. She had visited the day before and made a note that Mom did not look good, had lost a lot of weight and was very confused. In addition, her clothes were not clean, and her room was a mess.

July 23

I sent a document to the Couchiching Ontario Health Team (COHT) outlining the gaps in the Patient Caregiver Advisory Committee (PFAC). Due to the pandemic, we have not been successful at expanding the Committee beyond the Chair, currently occupied by me. I recommended that we restart the Advisory Committee once the Joint Executive Team (JET) decides on budget, structure, and accountability. According to the Provincial mandate, the PFAC needs a voice in the development of all Health Care Policies.

28 July

I had a conference call with the COHT. They agreed with my recommendations regarding the PFAC. I will now be a voting member of the JET. That is one more meeting for me to attend, but it is important, especially during the pandemic. The public needs a voice.

Remdesivir obtained approval from Health Canada for the treatment of COVID-19 patients. It was released as an Emergency Drug. I wondered how this affects the Emergency release of the COVID-19 vaccines.

July 31

A voluntary smartphone app that can warn you if you come into close proximity to someone who has tested positive for COVID-19 became available to download. I doubted very many would put it on their phone. They would probably consider it an infringement on their privacy.

Chapter 7
AUGUST 2020

August 3

The Canadian Football League cancelled its 2020 season.

August 5

I attended a JET conference call to discuss the PFAC policy documents I drafted.

A city councillor called to ask if the COHT would partner with Information Orillia and the Age-Friendly Orillia Advisory Committee in support of the Senior News program. I forwarded an email to the JET. When I received approval, I sent a letter confirming the support of the Orillia Seniors News line to the councillor. This will enable the city to obtain a provincial grant for the initiative.

August 11

I have an Operations and an Ethics Committee meeting today. They both sent documents for review prior to the meetings.

August 13

One of the JET members called and asked if I would be prepared to make the introductory remarks at the Couchiching Ontario Health

Team retreat on August 20. I agreed.

August 15

Our son called later that evening. They had to take our grandson for his COVID-19 screening test in preparation for his surgery on August 18. What an ordeal. The testing center was in a tent in the Alliston, Ontario, hospital parking lot, and it was poorly lit. When they drove in, their car was surrounded by technicians in full hazmat suits, which scared the poor five-year-old to death. Then they reached inside the car and held a long Q-Tip in front of his face and attempted to push it up his nose. He freaked out, so three people had to hold him down while he struggled and screamed, and they hurt his nose in the process. Poor little guy.

August 17

I drafted the Introductory Remarks for the COHT retreat and sent them to the JET for review.

August 20

I participated in the COHT strategy retreat via video. I made the introductory remarks as Chair of the PFAC. I raised concerns about the fact that dental, sight, hearing, chiropractic, physiotherapy, massage, and holistic medicine are not supported by the COHT. These services impact the overall health and wellbeing of individuals, especially vulnerable seniors, lower-income families and the homeless.

I also relayed a concern raised by the Indigenous community about losing seniors to COVID-19. It would result in a major loss of language and culture knowledge.

I recommended that the COHT obtain community feedback by conducting a survey.

Chapter 8

SEPTEMBER 2020

September 8

It is the first day of school tomorrow for our grandson. He is starting Grade one this year and is excited to see his friends again. He is one of hundreds of thousands of children and teenagers across the country to re-enter classrooms for the first time in six months.

Mom's retirement home has introduced a new visitor policy. They have hired a third party to aid with the increase in violence within the home. Their isolation rooms are now being used as "behaviour" rooms. Visitors must now book a visit with residents, and they must provide a minimum of forty-eight hours' notice. All visitors must wear masks and PPE when entering a resident's room, and no visitors or residents are allowed in the common areas.

September 14

The Canadian Bloc Québécois and Conservative parties declared self-isolation due to members infected with COVID-19.

September 16

I went to the Orillia Soldiers Memorial Hospital for my bone density scan. There have been a lot of changes made since the pandemic began. Outpatients coming to the hospital for tests and procedures may only enter by the front doors – no other entries are available. This means that long walks from the parking facilities are necessary. Patients are then screened for COVID-19 and made to change their personal masks for a new surgical mask. There are no longer volunteers available to direct patients to their destination. Patients must register by computer and then follow signs that direct them to the designated department. I really missed the personal touch.

The Canadian Federal Conservative Party leader, his family and some party members are in self-isolation after an aide tested positive for COVID-19.

September 18

The Nunavut territory in Canada reported its first cases of COVID-19.

September 22

I participated in a hospital Operations meeting:

The number of COVID-19 cases and tests is on the rise.

The hospital is preparing for a second wave.

The younger cohort makes up the majority of the infected, and they are less likely to require hospitalization.

The hospital staff is expecting a peak in November, like the flu virus, but not as bad as last spring.

The province has introduced gathering size reductions from twenty-five people to ten.

The Essential Visitor document has been drafted for patients and families.

The COVID-19 assessment center is struggling with people coming from other areas.

PPE supplies are at a critical level with only five to seven days' inventory.

The staff is worried that they may need to return to the March and April procedures.

A new drug for the treatment of severe cases has been approved for clinical trial by Health Canada. The Barrie Royal Victoria Hospital (RVH) is one of the approved sites. Patients from the Orillia Soldiers Memorial Hospital cannot be transferred to RVH due to a lack of beds. They may have access by late October.

We may need to revert to two meetings every week.

A friend called and discussed her meeting with her mom's Personal Support Worker (PSW). The PSW is overwhelmed with work and will not be able to help her any longer. She will need to care for her mom at home on her own.

September 23

PM Trudeau announced that the second wave of COVID-19 is underway. He said that Canadian families will probably not be able to gather for Thanksgiving this year.

September 25

Tougher restrictions have been reintroduced in Ontario.

September 29

A new daily high in COVID-19 cases was reported in Ontario yesterday. It reached over 700 cases.

I attended an Operations meeting. The hospital is planning to establish a bladder cancer treatment clinic using the BCG vaccine. BCG is short for Bacillus Calmette-Guerin, named after two French scientists who developed it from a weakened strain of Mycobacterium Bovis, a bacterium closely related to the one that causes M. tuberculosis (TB).

I told them that I was the person who managed the project at Connaught Laboratories Limited. I obtained Canadian and US regulatory approvals in 1990 for high-dose BCG as an immunotherapeutic product to treat some forms of bladder cancer. The special formulation of the company's BCG Vaccine was regulated as a therapeutic drug rather than as a vaccine and hence required additional clinical trials to look at long-term safety and duration of effect. I considered mentioning the type of clinical trials that should have been required for the mRNA COVID-19 vaccines, but resisted the temptation with difficulty.

September 30

The Canadian Federal government announced the launch of the Canadian Emergency Response Benefit (CERB) support program with a more "flexible and generous employment insurance regime than the Unemployment Insurance program." I do not understand why they need a new program rather than using the Unemployment Insurance program that people paid into and has been successfully running for decades.

Chapter 9
OCTOBER 2020

October 1

Stringent new rules take effect in Quebec for twenty-eight days. The rules include prohibiting private gatherings.

October 2

President Trump and his wife announced that they have Covid-19 and are self-isolating.

October 3

A couple from Etobicoke, Ontario just moved in across the street. They said that they needed to get away from Toronto because it has become difficult to live there since the pandemic. I think that they will be the first of many who will move out of the big cities over the coming months. It will drive the value of homes up and will make it difficult for locals to afford a house.

October 5

I spoke to the Orillia City councillor, who was a former reporter for our local paper, about my reading role for the Senior News Line. He said that I will need to prepare a summary of local news and limit the recording to a maximum of three minutes. I committed to two days every week and will focus on health news. I sent a clarification email to the project manager and the President of Information Orillia, who will host the Seniors News Line.

October 7

I prepared and recorded my first news broadcast:

"Dr. Gardner, Health Minister of Simcoe county, issues orders to enforce self-isolation rules.

Failure to comply with a self-isolation order could mean a fine of up to five thousand dollars per day.

The order takes effect October 6, 2020, and remains in effect until the Ministry of Health declares it is no longer needed.

The order applies to any person living or present in the County of Simcoe and District of Muskoka, Ontario, who diagnosed with Covid-19, has the signs and symptoms of Covid-19, has been tested for Covid-19 and is awaiting the results of their test, who has reasonable grounds to believe they have one or more symptoms of Covid-19, or who is a close contact of a person identified as a person diagnosed with Covid-19.

If you think you have any symptoms of Covid-19, use the Ontario provincial Covid-19 self-assessment tool, and if indicated by the tool, get tested and self-isolate at home for ten days (the period of time you are contagious) or until your test result is negative for

Covid-19.

If you have been identified as a close contact of someone with Covid-19, which means being within two metres of that infected person for at least fifteen minutes without adequate personal protective equipment (PPE), you must self-isolate for fourteen days even though you don't have symptoms.

Orillia's Covid-19 assessment centre moved from outside Soldiers Memorial Hospital to the Rotary Place on University Avenue, Orillia yesterday.

On Friday, the Ontario provincial government announced that assessment centres would only be open for appointments, discontinuing walk-in testing services.

Lab results are currently taking about five days to be returned.

Appointments should be made online. If you do not have access to the internet, a phone number is available to call to make an appointment, however, the phones are not always manned. Call 211 for more information.

Ontario confirms five hundred and forty-eight new Covid-19 cases today. The province has also confirmed seven new deaths today and reported five hundred and forty-six recoveries.

The latest fatalities have included one person between sixty and seventy-nine, and six people over the age of eighty. Two of the people who have died were residents at long-term care facilities.

Included in today's new cases are fourteen long-term care residents and nine health care workers.

There are currently fifty long-term care homes in outbreak with one hundred and twenty-four active cases in residents and one hundred and fifty-eight active cases in staff. There have been eight staff and eighteen hundred and seventy-three resident deaths attributed to the coronavirus reported since January.

UPDATE: sixteen residents and six staff Covid-19 cases confirmed at Simcoe Manor in Beeton, Ontario.

Long-term care home in Beeton sees twenty-two total cases of Covid-19 so far but is still waiting on test results for some staff and residents.

One person is dead and twenty-two cases of Covid-19 have been confirmed at Simcoe Manor, but the health unit has not yet determined how the virus got into the facility in the first place.

Two deaths occurred over the weekend at the facility. One, an eighty-eight-year-old man, has been confirmed as Covid-19 positive. The other person who died had been tested for Covid-19, but results have not yet come back as of Monday at 4 p.m. The test results are expected back in the next twenty-four to forty-eight hours.

The cause of transmission has not yet been determined.

Extensive protocols remain in place to stop the spread within the home.

Protocols include temporary cancellations of visitors (with some exceptions), enhanced cleaning measures, advanced screening, assigning staff to individual units during each shift and a temporary hold on all new resident admissions and internal transfers.

Staff are now required to wear full protective equipment, including gloves, gowns, masks and face shields upon entering units, and all residents are isolated in their rooms for precautionary reasons, with tray service for meals. Residents are using disposable plates, cups and cutlery for the duration of the outbreak to provide additional infection control safety.

The adjacent Simcoe Village is not in outbreak."

My husband and I watched the US Vice President debate between Kamala Harris and Mike Pence. Pence was so boring and lied so many times with a straight face that a fly landed on his head and stayed there for two minutes and twenty-three seconds. He didn't even notice. The internet went wild with memes.

October 8

The city councillor called and told me that I did a good job reading the news yesterday. He said that they added one more volunteer, so

I need only broadcast on Mondays beginning October 19. There is so much pandemic news to report, we agreed that I may exceed the three-minute limit if necessary.

October 10

Mom's nurse called us at 11:00 pm. Mom was sexually assaulted in her bed by a senior male resident. The police have been called, her door locked and the male resident has been detained.

I spoke to the police officer who asked if I wanted to press charges. I told him that it did not make sense that we press charges when the man who committed the crime was old and suffered with the same dementia as my mom. The officer said that he hoped I would see it the same way he did. I did tell him that we will investigate moving my mom to a more secure facility. He agreed that would be for the best and in the meantime the retirement home will be required to increase their security for vulnerable residents such as my mom. What makes this incident more concerning is the ability of residents to move from room to room, possibly spreading Covid-19.

October 11

I sent an email to mom's retirement home expressing our outrage and that we plan to move mom to a different Long Term Care facility in Orillia. I demanded that they keep mom's door always locked. It is not bad enough that mom must endure the hardships of the pandemic in her last years. She also must be subjected to sexual harassment. The lack of adequate staff to handle the additional responsibilities and visitor policies resulting from the pandemic is resulting in unsafe conditions for the vulnerable.

October 12

The president of the hospital sent me an email asking me to review a new government guideline and provide comments before the next JET meeting. It was a thirty-nine-page Ontario Health document titled Optimizing Care Through Covid-19 Transmission Scenarios.

October 13

I sent the following ethics scenario to the Operations Committee for discussion:

"The Orillia area is experiencing a significant increase in community Covid-19 cases. There are 3 Covid-19 patients currently in hospital and 1 patient died of Covid-19 complications 2 days earlier.

An Orillia resident enters the front entrance of the hospital not wearing a mask. When asked to put one of the hospital masks on they refuse, citing that the Covid-19 pandemic is a hoax.

The patient, who passes the oral screening and does not have a fever, has an appointment with the MRI department for a scan of his brain because he has been experiencing black outs. The diagnostic department is not happy receiving the patient without a mask. The hospital policy states that masks must be worn by everyone, including outpatients unless they have a medical reason put in writing by their physician. This patient did not have a valid exemption.

Should the patient be turned away if they refuse to wear a mask?"

After much discussion and support for turning the patient away, it was agreed that the mask policy would be amended to allow for exceptions. The final decision will rest with the referring physician.

As requested, I reviewed the Optimizing Care Through Covid-19 Transmission Scenarios. I then prepared a three-page summary and sent it to the hospital President in preparation for the next JET meeting. The summary included the following:

Throughout the document, "maintaining" services refer to continuing the existing levels of service without increasing or decreasing activities that will impact capacity. "Resuming" care refers to increasing services back to pre-pandemic levels, and "accelerating" services refer to increasing services above pre-pandemic levels to help alleviate the backlog of care deferred from previous waves of the pandemic.

The document included four recommendations:

Scenario one (no cases) will allow accelerating services.

Scenario two (sporadic cases) will allow resuming or accelerating services.

Scenario three (clusters of cases) will allow resuming services.

Scenario four (community transmission – moderate or widespread) will allow maintaining services.

I left a message on the Local Health Integration Network' (LHIN) answering machine about moving mom to a Long-Term Care home.

I have not yet received a response to my email to the Manager of mom's current facility.

October 14

I prepared and recorded my news update for the Senior News Line.

"There were no new cases reported in Orillia, however there are four people currently hospitalized in the region including one person from Orillia.

The region's health unit has confirmed fifty-three new Covid-19 cases in Simcoe County and two in Muskoka District since it last reported on Friday. The province reports:

The health unit is reporting sixteen new cases in Barrie, Ontario,

There are three new cases in Innisfil, Ontario,

There are fifteen new cases in Bradford West Gwillimbury,

There are eleven new cases in New Tecumseth,

There are two new cases in Essa County, and

The remaining four Simcoe County cases reported today include three women from Adjala-Tosorontio and one in Penetanguishene.

Two Muskoka cases include one in Muskoka county and one in the town of Bracebridge.

There were seven hundred and forty-six new Covid-19 cases in Ontario today and eight hundred and six yesterdays.

The Royal Victoria Regional Health Care in Barrie will temporarily manage Simcoe Manor following a provincial order.

Four residents have died at the long-term care home, which is operated by County of Simcoe; 'The province is using every tool available to keep Ontarians safe'

The Ministry of Long-Term Care announced today that it has issued a mandatory management order appointing Royal Victoria Regional Health Centre (RVH) to temporarily manage Simcoe Manor in Beeton on behalf of the County of Simcoe.

RVH has been managing Simcoe Manor since Friday, Oct. 9 after the Simcoe Muskoka District Health Unit issued an order under the Health Protection and Promotion Act.

RVH will manage Simcoe Manor for 90 days from the date that the mandatory management order was issued.

Simcoe Manor has one hundred and twenty-four residents, thirty-five of whom have tested positive for Covid-19. Additionally, nineteen staff members have also tested positive at the facility, according to new figures presented this morning at Simcoe County council.

Four residents have died, including an eighty-eight-year-old man, a ninety-two-year-old woman, a ninety-eight-year-old man, and an eighty-two-year-old woman.

The Couchiching Pharmacist Network has been collaborating with local health-care providers to ensure everyone is vaccinated for the upcoming flu season.

The standard dose vaccine is available for everyone over the age of 5. It is a quadrivalent vaccine, which will protect against four different strains of influenza.

If you are 65 or older, you can receive either the standard dose, or high dose vaccine. The high dose flu shot is a trivalent vaccine which contains three strains of influenza, just in higher concentrations.

The high dose vaccine is usually reserved for vulnerable at-risk seniors, such as those with autoimmune conditions. However, either vaccine is a safe and effective choice for generally healthy seniors. Getting one flu shot is enough for the year, and booster doses are not recommended.

Many pharmacies will now require an appointment for a flu shot. Some will have designated hours for walk-in traffic. This will help manage the workflow in the pharmacy, and give staff time to ensure enough supplies, complete the necessary screening and cleaning measures.

Pharmacies are in the early stages of receiving an initial vaccine supply. Current available appointments may be limited by the preliminary release of supply, but increased quantities will be more available in the coming weeks.

Rapid Covid-19 tests coming to provinces and territories 'shortly'.

The Prime Minister of Canada confirmed today that the federal government is continuing to provide surge support on processing tests and boosting testing capacity in response to Covid-19

Orillia City secures emergency Covid-19 funding for Leacock Museum

According to a memo to city councillors, the grant will be used to help "offset lost revenue at the museum resulting from temporary closures and new protocols that limit visitors to the property to help stop the spread of Covid-19."

The memo notes "the museum has taken important steps to create a safe and welcoming experience for all. This includes pre-registration, staggered entry for individual social circles, hand sanitizing stations and touchless payment in the gift shop."

Visitors can also download the self-guided tour of the house to their mobile device. Guests can book an exclusive time for their social circle (up to five people) to tour the house Monday to Friday between 12 p.m. and 3 p.m., exclusive of holidays. "

Judy from the LHIN called me about mom's situation. We will meet in mom's room next Wednesday, October 21 to discuss next steps while we are waiting for a LTC vacancy.

The President of Orillia Soldiers Memorial Hospital emailed me with a request to speak this afternoon to the JET about my review of the government scenario document.

I could not reach mom this morning. There is still no response to my email from the Manager. At 10:30 am the manager called me and said that she placed a sign on mom's door with instructions to keep it locked. I thanked her and requested she put her action in writing. She declined.

The meeting coordinator of the COHT called and we discussed tomorrow's COHT meeting and my PFAC and Covid-19 updates.

October 15

I participated in the COHT meeting and spoke about the Covid-19 scenario recommendations provided by Ontario Health. I also spoke about the restart of the PFAC.

October 16

The constable who is handling mom's sexual assault case called to discuss what happened and to tell me that due to the degree of dementia of both parties, no charges will be laid. He will follow up with the management to ensure that their recommendations were followed.

October 19

I prepared and recorded my script for the News Line.

"The new Covid-19 assessment centre at Rotary Place 'running very well'

Two weeks ago, it was not uncommon for people to be idling in their vehicles, waiting for up to five hours to get a Covid-19 test at the drive-through assessment centre at Orillia Soldiers Memorial Hospital.

But since the assessment centre has moved to the Rotary Place and transitioned to an appointment-only service, people can get their tests now in less than a half hour.

The assessment centre is open from 11:00 am to 6:30 pm Monday to Friday, and from 11:00 am to 2:30 pm on weekends and holidays.

Appointments should be booked online.

Appointments can also be booked by calling the centre.

211 information services provide 'great value' for local residents

The service includes information and referral specialists, 24/7, call centre services available in multiple languages, and emergency management,

Orillia Provincial Offences Court will stay closed until January 22. Those impacted will be sent a new court date via mail."

Canada's Covid-19 case count surpassed 200,000 today. This is double the number reported four months ago.

October 20

I have an Operations meeting at noon, and a new committee meeting called PFAC Network at 6:00 pm. The latter is a network of all Patient Family Advisory Committees in Ontario. As Chair of the Patient Caregiver Advisory Committee (PFAC) for the Couchiching Ontario Health Team and a member of the Orillia Hospital Patient Family Advisory Committee I was selected to represent the Couchiching region. This is a volunteer position requiring several hours every week.

During the PFAC Network meeting, I suggested a cross-fertilization of the LHIN and OHT PFAC's. There are so many acronyms, it is hard to keep track. Hopefully my senior brain will not fail me any time soon. I have too many projects on the go and so many people relying on me.

October 21

I went to meet with the LHIN representative and mom about the move to a LTC facility. I selected my five top choices of LTC facilities in the Orillia area and included them on the application form. The LHIN put mom on the Ontario LTC crisis list, the highest priority category for people whose safety is a significant risk without prompt LTC placement. This includes those unable to be cared for at home, hospital patients blocking beds during hospital crisis or community cases lacking support. Currently the normal wait time is 4-5 years. Hopefully, the crisis list will mean an earlier move. The only downside of being on the crisis list is we must accept the first bed offered or risk losing priority.

October 22

Mom's physician came to our house planning to give her a flu shot. I told him that mom did not live with us and did not want to receive any vaccines. She had a bad reaction last time she received an annual flu shot.

It was a good thing that he came to my home rather than going directly to the retirement home. He would have administered the vaccine, and we would have not known about it. We discussed the "assault incident" and reasons for me wanting to move her as quickly as possible. I gave him a copy of the LHIN transfer application, and he will sign it today. We recognize that he will not be her doctor once she moves to another facility.

October 28

A report from Canada's chief medical officer said that Canada ranks twenty-sixth in the world for total deaths per million populations. That is rather hard to believe considering the level of precaution in Canada. Most of the deaths in Canada occur in hospitals or LTC homes. Very few deaths are reported outside hospitals. I wonder why that is? Is it because everyone who advances to serious disease is admitted to hospital or is it because the treatment protocols used in the hospitals are causing deaths? It would be interesting to know what treatment protocols are being used in the countries with lowest death rates.

October 31

Due to the pandemic, kids will not be allowed to go out trick or treating this year. I feel so sorry for the little ones who do not understand why they are prevented from seeing their family and friends, going to school and participating in sports.

Chapter 10

NOVEMBER 2020

November 2

I prepared and recorded the health news for tomorrow.

Ontario confirms 977 new Covid-19 cases today as well as 864 recoveries and 9 deaths.

The 9 new deaths include 3 people between the ages of 60 and 79 years old, and 6 people over the age of 80. Four of the people who died were residents at long-term care homes.

November 5

At 9:30 am the US Presidential election counts for Joe Biden are at 263 and Donald Trump's are at 214. They are still counting and recounting.

November 7

At noon, CNN called Biden the winner of the Presidential election. Everyone we know is happy with the result.

November 9

It was becoming hard to keep track of all the volunteer work I am currently involved in, so I made a list and filled a calendar full of meetings.

Orillia Soldiers Memorial Hospital, member of the –

Operations Committee,

Patient and Family Advisory Committee, and

Ethics Committee.

Couchiching Ontario Health Team, member of the –

Joint Executive Team, voting member,

Collaboration Table,

Patient Caregiver Advisory Committee, Chair,

Patient Family Advisory Committee Network, Rotating Chair.

Repair Café – Tom and I repair broken items free of charge.

City Sunshine Initiative – involved in several projects including the Senior News Line.

November 11

Today is a day for Remembrance. There will not be a Remembrance Day ceremony this year.

I listened to one of the volunteers who called to complain about how her mom was treated when she was admitted into the hospital from the Emergency Department. She was taken to the emergency department a few days before and was diagnosed with a serious heart condition. Her mom has dementia, so they had to restrain her. My friend is not allowed to visit more than a couple of hours every day, and once she leaves is not permitted to return until the next day. She is considering taking her mom home and managing herself. Although it will be extremely difficult, she said it was preferable to the current conditions in the hospital.

I will use this example to provide comments and suggestions for improvement during the next hospital Operations Committee meeting.

November 15

I prepared and recorded the news report for tomorrow:

"The number of cases in Canada has reached 300,000. That is an increase in 100,000 cases in the past month.

Ontario reports 1248 new Covid-19 cases today and 29 deaths.

The number of deaths being reported today in Ontario is the highest in a single day since June.

A recent poll says fifteen percent of Canadians are skeptical about Covid-19 risks.

The majority of Canadians are aware of the public health risk of Covid-19, but a high percent say they don't believe the virus poses a big health risk to the general population.

The findings raised questions among public health experts about how to address those who don't believe in the seriousness of a virus that has killed more than 10,000 Canadians, and whether their skepticism poses a risk as Covid-19 cases continue to rise at a high rate.

At the time the survey was conducted, Covid-19 cases reached unprecedented highs in Toronto and Ontario. On Wednesday, Ontario broke another daily record with more than 1400 cases reported.

The health experts believe that it's unlikely that the opinion of Covid-19 non-believers will change. The solution then lies in sidestepping the problem by implementing mandatory mask-wearing and other simple, effective measures.

For those who are worried, people should focus on what is within their own control: following safety measures, staying informed, preparing for the unpredictability of the virus and reaching out for help when it's needed."

I do not think the survey results are accurate and disagree with the government's classification of "non-believers" and their proposed solution of mandates. Healthy younger people and children are not at risk of severe disease and typically do not worry about the annual influenza outbreaks. Most recover quickly without any long-term effects. The reports of deaths in the news are mainly in the elderly and individuals with other existing health problems, such as lung disease, obesity, heart disease or diabetes. The risk of infection in these groups can be reduced by avoidance of exposure. Everyone else can get on with their lives as they do during the influenza season.

November 16

Canada's case count exceeds 300,000, less than a month since the count was 200,000.

November 17

I participated in the Operations meeting. The team appeared very stressed. After the meeting, I sent information about time management courses to the Director and external psychology support for the staff.

November 18

I joined the Ethics Committee meeting today, reviewed the Ethics Toolkit after the meeting and emailed comments to the Chair.

November 19

The private nurse I hired to trim mom's nails, made a note on her recent invoice that said mom was very confused and had lost more weight.

I participated in a COHT meeting. There is so much happening in the area, we spent much of the meeting deciding what takes priority.

November 22

I prepared and recorded today's health news-

"Simcoe Muskoka is moving into the province's orange "restrict" level for a minimum of twenty-eight days, with further control measures in place to prevent the spread of Covid-19.

Under the orange restrictions all restaurants and food and drink establishments must close by 10 p.m. and stop serving alcohol by 9:00 p.m. A maximum of four people may be seated together, and there cannot be more than fifty people seated indoors.

Sports and recreational facilities are limited to fifty people per facility, and the fitness/lesson class capacity is still capped at ten people. No spectators are permitted except for parents and guardians for the supervision of children.

Personal care services including steam rooms, saunas, whirlpools, floating pools and sensory deprivation pods must close. Services requiring the removal of face coverings are prohibited. Contact your caregiver for more information.

All indoor visits at long-term care homes in the region will be limited to one essential visitor at a time.

As Covid-19 cases surge, a Regional Pandemic Response Unit opens in Barrie

The seventy-bed, fully equipped field hospital in the parking lot of

Barrie's RVH is a four-season, tented structure intended as an overflow for hospitals throughout the region as the pandemic persists and puts pressure on the medical sector.

The temporary unit will operate indefinitely and is intended to serve not just patients going to RVH, but also those seeking medical attention at hospitals in Alliston, Collingwood, Georgian Bay, Orillia and Muskoka Algonquin.

It is not a Covid-19 unit. The patients who will be cared for here are medically stable with an estimated stay of three to five days. This will create room in the main hospitals for Covid-19 patients.

One last bit of health news

New evidence indicates that wearing a well-fitting face mask made with a minimum of two layers, each of a different material, and keeping a six feet distance also protects the wearer as well as those around them. Avoiding in-door contact with those not living with you has also been shown to reduce the spread of disease."

November 24

I participated in the Ethics Framework workshop today from 11:00 am to 1:00 pm. The meeting went well except I lost my internet connection in the middle of my presentation. I finished giving my report ten minutes later. Relying on the internet for meetings during the pandemic has been a major problem for me.

November 25

Our new next-door neighbour dropped off a lovely Christmas wreath his wife made for us. She suffers with Louie Body Dementia and aphasia. I stayed with her occasionally when her husband needed to go out for appointments or shopping. She was a nurse by profession and understood the risk I took during the pandemic. The wreath was her way of showing her appreciation and I was touched by her thoughtfulness. We proudly mounted it to our exterior wall next to the front door for all to see.

I participated in the Provincial PFAC meeting –

A new Ombudsman for Patients was appointed by the Premier. They will be involved in LTC, hospitals, home and community care as managed by the LHIN. Patients or families must first go to the point of care. The Ombudsman is the office of last resort.

The Ombudsman is not the same as a patient advocate who look for fairness for both the patient and the healthcare workers.

The greatest number of complaints received by the Ombudsman will be from LTC and hospitals.

Studies determined that dementia patients do not benefit from virtual visits.

We reviewed the essential visitor protocols and will put forward the following recommendations:

Backstops for all healthcare workers

Change the visitation protocol

Ensure dedicated communication resources

Ensure whistleblower protection.

Essential visitors compared to partners in care was discussed.

The allowance of visits by patients' essential care givers is a requirement. However, there is no requirement for hospitals or LTC homes to advertise that requirement. I understood that this meant that the public is unaware of their rights.

After the meeting I sent an email to our hospital asking that the hospital's website be updated to include this information about essential caregivers and that patient families be informed about this exception when the patient is admitted.

I also spoke to mom's management about designating me as an essential caregiver and followed it up with an email. I wish that I had known this earlier. It is another example of "lies by omission".

November 26

Trudeau announced that Canada has purchase agreements with seven Covid-19 vaccine producers.

Mom's home sent me forms to sign to become her essential caregiver and allow me to visit with conditions. I may go afternoons any day except Wednesdays.

November 27

I am remembering dad's ninety-eighth birthday today. He has been gone fourteen years, and I have been my mom's caregiver since he left us. Mom is now ninety-six. It is unfortunate that she is living through the horrors of the pandemic.

I visited mom and she was in bed and mumbling when I arrived. I do not think that she knew it was me. The room looks like a bomb went off. I spent forty-five minutes organizing and cleaning her room. Tomorrow I will organize her dresser drawers.

Trudeau said that most Canadians should receive the Covid-19 vaccine by September 2021. Vaccine distribution will be led by the former NATO commander.

November 29

I prepared and recorded the news –

"Council approved 20,000 dollars to help attract newcomers to Orillia.

During operating budget discussions last week, city councillors voted to allocate twenty thousand dollars to create "newcomer packages" and incentives to help persuade people to move to Orillia.

The decision is subject to ratification at a special meeting of council December 7.

The idea is a "staff initiative" that stemmed from conversations with Hydro One officials.

"They are moving hundreds of employees" to their new facility in west Orillia and the city would like those employees to move to Orillia.

This initiative would provide about one hundred dollars' worth of incentives to each newcomer.

Newcomers would receive one-time discount vouchers to city-owned facilities, including the Orillia Recreation Centre, Orillia Opera House, Leacock Museum as well as for transit and parking."

I did some research about dementia patients and bought mom a life-like baby doll yesterday. I spent the morning organizing baby clothes to use with it.

Mom was sitting in her wheelchair today. She was non-responsive until I gave her the doll to hold. I told her she needed to take care of it for me. She then came to life, although she did not know who I was. When I left, she was still sitting in the chair hugging the doll. I spoke to the staff and explained what I had done and they thought it was an excellent idea. I suggested that they purchase some dolls for other residents suffering from dementia. I plan to donate a few and ask that they give them to the few residents I knew personally.

Chapter 11 – DECEMBER 2020

December 1

As requested by the Operations Committee, I reviewed the plans for the new CT scan suite at the hospital. I sent them comments about personnel and equipment flow.

Today, I started working on my memoir focusing on my career at Connaught Labs. I spent twenty years there from 1972 to 1992. During those years, there were so many major events that I was involved in, such as the evolution of the regulatory agencies, the AIDS epidemic, the blood scandal, the Ebola epidemic, approval of BCG vaccine as an immunotherapeutic for bladder cancer, the sale of the only Canadian vaccine manufacturer to the French, the introduction of influenza and meningococcal vaccines in Canada, the development failure of an AIDs vaccine, Polio vaccine recalls and shortage, insulin improvements, and the evolution of the computer age.

December 2

Johnson and Johnson began the process of applying for emergency approval of its Covid-19 vaccine from Health Canada. Pfizer has been given permission to release its Covid-19 vaccine for emergency use in the UK. The news articles did not explain the difference between Emergency Approval and full approval. Most people will think that the vaccines are similar to influenza vaccines and that their approval is based on all the safety testing required by the regulations. The government led by omission to deceive the public into thinking that they are our saviour, and that the vaccines are the solution to stopping the pandemic.

December 4

Canada recorded more than 400,000 cases, just eighteen days after 300,000 was reached.

December 7

I prepared and recorded the news-

“Some promising stories in the Covid-19 news today:

Rapid testing at Soldiers allows more ‘reactive’ response to Covid-19

In thirteen minutes, you could have the results of your Covid-19 test.

It’s been about three weeks since Orillia Soldiers was one of several hospitals across Ontario selected for the rapid testing pilot project. The project was intended to provide rapid tests to more rural areas of Ontario to control spread of Covid-19.

The test is taken in the same way as a regular Covid-19 test, through a nasal swab, but the results come back within thirteen minutes and are processed at the hospital. Regular Covid-19 tests need to be sent to a lab in Toronto for processing, which is what can lead to delays in getting results.

Once results come back from the rapid test, patients are still recommended to follow up with a traditional test. The purpose of the rapid test is to stop potential spread as quickly as possible and aid in contact tracing.

For the time being rapid tests can only be used for symptomatic health-care workers, in-patients with symptoms and asymptomatic individuals who have had direct contact with a Covid-19 case.

The other use is in congregate living facilities, or other facilities where there's potential for an outbreak.

Barrie's RVH agrees to store Covid-19 vaccine when available

The federal government announced last week that the newly approved Pfizer's Covid-19 vaccine will arrive and could be administered to a target group as early as this week with a plan to vaccinate the general population beginning April to the end of 2021.

The provincial government announced Friday that phase one of its roll-out plan will see ninety thousand doses designated for health care workers in up to fourteen hospitals in grey and red areas first.

That news came just two hours after the province declared Simcoe-Muskoka would become a red zone starting Monday. It's unclear if that means this area will be among those receiving the vaccine first."

My research uncovered that the rapid test is non-specific for the Covid-19 virus, so it has a very high false-positive rate. This will cause problems in the healthcare system due to the requirement to self-isolate for fourteen days after a positive test and will put a strain on the hospital where there already is a staffing issue.

December 8

The news reported that partial early results published in the Lancet suggest the Astra Zeneca Covid-19 vaccine is "safe and seventy percent effective". I reviewed the publication and noted that the trial did not monitor recipients beyond three months and did not demonstrate protection against infection or spread.

December 9

I prepared and recorded the Health News:

"Today, December 9, Health Canada announced they have authorized the first Covid-19 vaccine. The application was received on October 9, 2020.

Health Canada stated in their announcement that after an independent and thorough scientific review, the vaccine meets the stringent safety, efficacy, and quality requirements for use in Canada. As part of their openness and transparency, they will release summary documents that support the release.

They also stated that Canadians can feel confident that the review process was rigorous and that we have a strong monitoring system."

The vaccine was authorized under Health Canada's new (September 16, 2020) Interim Order Respecting Importation, Sale and Advertising Drugs for Use in Relation to Covid-19. This order states that if the Minister of Health believes that an immediate action is required to deal with a significant risk, direct or indirect, to health, safety or environment a drug may be released for sale in Canada.

The US is using their similar Emergency Release regulation to approve Covid-19 vaccines.

Although I recorded the news as stated by the main news sources, I did not believe a word of what was written. Again, they lied by omission. The virus was isolated in January 2020. The time required to:

create a vaccine,

manufacture the vaccine,

perform early safety testing,

start the clinical trial patient recruitment,

monitor the patients for Covid-19 infection and long-term side effects compared to a placebo,

analyze the trial data,

gather data about the manufacture and testing of the vaccine batches for the trial and for mass distribution, and

prepare the submission to the regulators,

is impossible to complete by October 2020, which is only eight months from identification of the virus to submission of all the results.

Two of the vaccines were produced using a mRNA platform. When the release announcement was made, I discovered that they had changed the classification of the mRNA delivery system from a "gene therapy" to a "vaccine". This removed several safety and efficacy requirements. To add insult to injury, in September 2020, just one month before the vaccine submission, they created an Emergency Release regulation which exempted the "vaccine" from informed consent, product recall and liability.

In May, when Trump announced that a Covid-19 vaccine would be made available in January 2021 as part of Operation Warp Speed, I was skeptical. Now I am angry. These vaccines are experimental at best, and at a very early stage of development. To be fair, Trump said that the program was created to expedite development, manufacture and distribution of the new vaccines. He did not say anything about testing for safety or effectiveness. Again, the government lied by omission.

I called my son and warned them not to take the vaccine if it is made available to his age group. The issue is not that I know that the vaccine is unsafe, the issue is that there is no information that the vaccine is either safe or that it will prevent infection. An injection of something with no safety or effectiveness data into young healthy individuals is a crime. He agreed that he would let me know if they decide they needed to get vaccinated.

At this point, I will not believe anything the government says. I will have to do my own research and communicate my findings on social media and to the committees I am working with.

December 13

I prepared and recorded the Health News:

Trudeau announced that the first 30,000 doses of vaccine arrived in Canada today. He said that "the vaccine is expected to bring the outbreak to an end and the eventual return to normalcy. The vaccine must be stored at very low temperatures making movement difficult. Therefore, the first doses will be going to front line health care workers, employees and residents of long-term care homes in red zones.

The Pfizer vaccine will be going to long term care workers and Moderna will go to residents of long-term care in red zones.

Full protection requires two doses and will take twenty-eight days after the first dose. Everyone needs to continue to follow distancing, masking and hand washing until they are fully protected by the vaccine."

I do not understand how Trudeau can claim that the vaccine is expected to bring the outbreak to an end and that we can turn to normalcy. The clinical trials did not demonstrate that the vaccine stops infection or spread. The manufacturer only examined how many people were hospitalized due to Covid-19. In addition, they only studied the effects of the vaccine for three months. That was not sufficient time to determine if the vaccine protected from infection or if there were long-term effects from the vaccine. The placebo group were given the vaccine after three months so there was no opportunity to compare the two groups beyond that limited three months. Again, the government lied by omission.

December 14

The first doses of the Pfizer vaccine in Canada will be administered to people in Quebec and Ontario.

After dinner, my husband's youngest sister called and chatted for over an hour. Her and her husband are going stir crazy. They are so used to travelling and dining in restaurants. They have not been able to do either since the pandemic started and they have had no visitors. They both work from home, so they can still earn a living. They cannot wait to get the vaccine. I started to discuss my concerns, and I was told they did not want to hear about them. At first, I took it personally and then I realized that they were desperate to get their life back and they did not want to hear anything that would prevent it. I fear that is going to be the attitude of most people.

December 15

I prepared and recorded the Health News:

“Trudeau announced again that “Phase one of vaccine roll-out will begin with front-line Health Care workers. The vaccine has been approved by Health Canada and is ready for administration.”

“As more doses arrive, they will ensure that every person who wants a vaccine will receive one. While vaccines will not be mandatory, everyone will be encouraged to receive it.”

Trudeau stated that “Health Canada authorized the vaccine after an independent and thorough scientific review for safety, effectiveness and quality. Health Canada will continue to monitor for safety and effectiveness”.

Health Canada may have conducted a “thorough scientific review”, but they had very little information to review. They obviously did not ask questions or request additional information. There was not sufficient time for the companies to generate more data or information to respond to deficiencies if Health Canada did ask questions.

At least, the government is only offering the vaccine to those who want it. They are not forcing individuals to get it. That means that if people do their homework, healthy young people and children will not receive the experimental drug. That makes me feel a bit better about the government's deceit.

I spent an hour with the Operations team at noon. They are preparing to vaccinate their staff. The relief felt during the meeting was palpable. I did not have an opportunity to outline my concerns.

I attended the JET meeting for one hour beginning at 5:30 pm. I raised my concerns about the vaccine and was told that the government would not allow it to be administered to people if it was not safe. In other words, shut up and mind my own business.

December 16

As the Chair of the PFAC, I was asked to send a letter of support to Age Friendly Orillia to include in their grant application.

December 17

I received a letter from mom's LTC home. It was addressed to Essential Caregivers and stated:

"We are in the Red Zone and there are several outbreaks currently in several homes in the region.

Conditions include weekly Covid-19 tests and proof of negative result.

Surgical masks to be worn correctly the entire time with no exceptions. Non-compliance will result in revocation of essential caregiver status.

The resident must wear a mask the entire time.

Only the caregiver and resident are allowed in the room. No one else will be allowed.

Physical distancing must be followed. "

The last COHT meeting of the year was this afternoon. I did not raise any concerns at the meeting. Because patients will not receive vaccine over the holidays, I will wait until the new year to outline the issues.

I booked my first Covid-19 screening test for tomorrow. I must now get tested every Friday and send proof of negative results to mom's retirement home management before I can visit the following week. This does not make any sense to me, but I will not say anything because I do not want to be subjected to daily testing.

December 18

I went to have the Covid-19 test performed. I was impressed with the set up and efficiency when I walked into the arena. I was not impressed with the test. It really hurt and continued hurting for over two hours. I now know why our grandson screamed and struggled. I am not looking forward to getting it done every week.

December 20

Canada reached 500,000 cases. The federal government restricted travel from the UK for seventy-two hours to keep a highly contagious new strain of Covid-19 out of Canada.

December 21

I prepared and recorded the health news –

"BREAKING News:

All regions in the province of Ontario will be placed into grey-lockdown stage starting 12:00 am Christmas Eve.

The move will restrict non-essential retail and prohibit indoor dining right across the province.

The lockdown is expected to be in place for twenty-eight days in many regions, though the lockdown is expected to be only two weeks in the north.

Ford is expected to announce additional measures in a press conference today Monday at 1:00 p.m.

As part of the province's Coronavirus Response Framework, restrictions as part of the grey-lockdown level include a ban on indoor social gatherings with anyone that is not a part of your household, the closing of non-essential businesses as well as many fitness facilities, while restaurants and bars would be limited to takeout service only."

December 22

My Covid-19 test came back negative and I emailed the result to mom's home.

I participated in the Operations meeting and there was very little discussion about the vaccine.

December 23

Health Canada said that the Covid-19 vaccine from Moderna is safe to use in Canada. I am so disillusioned with the lack of transparency and the lies told by the government.

Just like the Pfizer vaccine, Moderna's vaccine is a mRNA product that makes cells produce spike protein and has limited safety data. The mRNA platform was never intended to be a vaccine. It was developed to treat malignant tumors. Dr. Malone, who was the original developer many years ago, has publicly stated that the mRNA technology is not safe as a vaccine. The government called him a conspiracy theorist who is spreading misinformation. His Facebook, Twitter and LinkedIn accounts were taken down by those platforms. This is what happens when you tell the truth. I will now need to be selective about the way I communicate my concerns.

December 25

It snowed last night so we have a lovely white Christmas.

Our son and grandson called us by video at 9:30 am. They showed us the inside of their new house in Barrys Bay and the live evergreen tree they decorated. Thank goodness for technology. We did not need to miss seeing their smiling faces today.

December 26

Ontario confirmed two cases of a more contagious variant of Covid-19 from the UK. The province is also re-entering a lockdown that prohibits non-essential business and closes all schools for at least two weeks.

December 28

Canada recorded over 15,000 Covid-19 deaths.

December 30

Air travellers must test negative for Covid-19 before landing in Canada.

December 31

It is the last day of 2020. We are so happy to see the back of it.

Chapter 12 – JANUARY 2021

January 3

Canada recorded 600,000 Covid-19 cases.

I went to visit mom and while I was there, one of the senior PSWs spoke to me in the hallway. She told me all about the problems they were having during the pandemic. Many of the residents' health declined significantly due to lack of socialization, visits from families, dehydration, malnourishment and isolation. There have been several deaths, none were due to Covid-19. The staff are exhausted and cannot cope with the amount of work without family assistance. She said that I was the only one visiting and they could see the improvement in mom's condition since I started coming in. The main reason people will not visit is due to the requirement for weekly Covid-19 screening. Most families of the residents do not live in Orillia and work during the week. They refuse to have the Covid-19 screening test done just to visit for 2 hours on weekends. I told her I am willing to do anything it takes to continue visiting my mom.

January 5

I attended an Operations meeting this morning. During the meeting, we reviewed the Covid-19 vaccine information sheet. The main points included in the document provided by the District Health Unit were -

It is not recommended that the following people be vaccinated -

pregnant, want to become pregnant or are breastfeeding,

have an autoimmune disorder, a weakened immune system, or severe allergies to anything requiring an epi pen.

People who have recovered from Covid-19 should still get the vaccine because natural immunity may not last very long. I speculated that natural immunity will last longer than any antibodies to the vaccine.

People still need to wear a mask, practice distancing and wash hands often until it is known if the vaccine prevents the spread of Covid-19 infections.

The information sheet is consistent with the information in the Product Monograph approved by Health Canada. However, it is not consistent with the information promoted by the government and health agencies. The government stated the vaccine is safe in all groups, including pregnant women. The government stated that the vaccine will end the pandemic. There are no data to support their claims that the vaccines protect against infection or spread.

I am disappointed that the medical community is not questioning the lies that are circulating. I can only assume that it is not malicious and that they are just too overwhelmed with the pandemic to question anything. It is up to people like me, who have no skin in the game, to educate them.

As I was leaving mom's home, the nurse at the front desk offered me the Covid-19 vaccine. I told her that due to my autoimmune conditions I should not receive it. I thanked her and told her to put a note in my mom's chart that she also cannot receive it. Her look was enough to indicate that she was shocked by my response and was not happy with my decision.

The staff and residents at retirement homes and LTC homes are the first to receive the vaccine after the front-line health care workers and first responders. They and their families feel a sense of relief and do not have the capacity or knowledge to question the government directives. Rather, they are grateful to the government for providing protection from this terrible disease. Little do they know that the vaccine may not protect them and that they may experience serious or long-term effects from it.

January 6

We are watching the US Senate meeting with protesters storming the Capital. After stirring them up, Trump was at his podium telling them to go home.

January 7

Last night, the US Senate voted and confirmed Biden for President.

I visited Mom today. She was complaining about pain, and I discovered that she has several bed sores. I called the nurse to clean and dress the sores. I will bring some ointment next time I come. Again, why do I have to instruct the staff about patient care. I do not want to think about the other residents and how worse off they are.

January 8

We woke to a winter wonderland. The sky is dark blue. The trees are covered in ice and sparkling in bright sunshine. Snow is falling in the absence of clouds. It reminds me of the Beatles song Lucy in the Sky with Diamonds. Some days I wish I could get some "Lucy."

Another new variant that first surfaced in South Africa was reported in Canada. The first vaccines used a spike protein isolated from the original Covid-19 virus to cause the body to develop an immune response. Any new variant would have a different spike protein. Therefore, the original vaccine would not be effective against new variants. By the time everyone who wants the vaccine gets it, the new variants will have replaced the original strain. This is why a vaccine for the common cold has never been developed. Adenoviruses, which cause the common cold, also quickly mutate. This is also why vaccinating the masses during a pandemic is not advisable. It may result in frequent mutations of the virus, producing more contagious and lethal strains. This is the result of vaccines that do not stop infection or spread.

January 11

I prepared and recorded the news.

"Few of us are likely to forget 2020.

But what about the next twelve months?

Other than overcoming the Covid-19 pandemic, community leaders say there is much in store for 2021.

The coming year represents a milestone and a new beginning for the Lighthouse, the non-profit organization that provides shelter and nourishment to Orillia's homeless. The Lighthouse will open the doors in late spring on a community-services hub featuring an emergency shelter for men, women, families and youths, with accompanying support services. Twenty supportive-housing units are also being constructed at the Queen Street site.

The Sharing Place Food Centre continues to see strong demand for services among members of the community struggling to survive. It is anticipated that the numbers will increase significantly as more people lose their jobs. A major focus will be to create a commercial kitchen to produce ready-made meals out of the facility for people that that have no fixed address or live in rooming houses that don't have fully equipped kitchens. The Dufferin Street operation expects to complete their renovation of the facility by spring.

A Covid-19 outbreak was declared at the Barrie hospital

Seven patients and two staff tested positive for coronavirus

Yesterday, Ontario reported another record 3,945 new Covid-19 cases and 61 deaths

Of the 3945 cases, 85 are from Simcoe-Muskoka.

Four of the deaths reported were individuals between 40 and 59 years old, eighteen were between 60 and 79, thirty-eight were over the age of 80.

As of 8 p.m. on Jan. 9, the province reported over 113,000 doses of vaccine have been administered and over 5000 individuals received the two required doses given twenty-one days apart.

There are more than 1100 active, lab-confirmed cases of Covid-19 in the region, with the majority of those in Simcoe County. At least 28 people from Simcoe County are currently hospitalized.

The Ontario government has implemented a province-wide shut down.

January 12

Ontario reported over 5000 Covid-19 deaths.

January 13

Another lockdown begins tonight at midnight.

One of the hospital volunteers called. She just found out that she needs surgery for advanced throat cancer and she has no idea when or where it will be done. She became the primary caregiver for her mom at home when she decided to remove her from the unacceptable hospital conditions. When her mother passed away at home a few weeks ago, she was able to see a doctor. She is under considerable stress, and stress is known to accelerate cancer.

January 14

I went for my weekly Covid-19 screening test, and it still hurts as much as the first time.

A stay-at-home order took effect in Ontario after 4000 daily cases were reported. The order also requires masks be worn inside businesses and the size of gatherings is restricted.

January 15

I was up early to prepare for a JET meeting at 8:00 am. After the meeting, one of the senior staff members called to discuss my mask and visitor recommendations. She agreed but said that the hospital will continue to follow government orders.

Pfizer reported stopping delivery of Covid-19 vaccine to Canada because of issues with production. They had scaled up their batch size after the clinical trials were completed on small pilot batches. Hopefully, the regulators required equivalency testing to be performed before allowing these batches on the market. I doubt that would be the case because there was not sufficient time to conduct more clinical testing.

One of the PFAC volunteers called me after dinner. She was concerned that the executives at the hospital were not listening to the hospital Patient and Family Advisory Committee. I sent an email to the PFAC coordinator about the issues the volunteer raised during our call. He responded that we would chat on Monday.

January 16

Today, Canada reported 700,000 Covid-19 cases.

January 18

I prepared and recorded the news.

"There is much confusion around the screening conducted by the Hospital prior to elective diagnostic procedures. When you arrive at the front entrance of the hospital you will be asked the following questions:

Do you have a fever, new cough, worsening cough or difficulty breathing?

Does anyone in your household have any of these symptoms?

Have you come in close contact with anyone with severe respiratory illness?

Have you travelled outside Canada in last fourteen days?

Do you have Covid-19 or had close contact with someone with Covid-19?

Do you have any one of the following symptoms: sore throat, chills, loss of taste or smell, nausea, vomiting, diarrhea, pink eye, runny nose or nasal congestion?

If you answer yes to any one of the above questions or symptoms, or if you refuse to wear a hospital mask, your entry into the hospital may be denied and your doctor contacted for further instructions which may include a test for Covid-19, postponing the procedure, or submitting a new urgent request.

If you have an appointment, you should avoid any of the listed situations. If you develop any of the symptoms, you should contact your referring physician.

These restrictions are in place to keep both patients and staff safe from Covid-19 infection. As a result, the hospital is one of the safest places in town. Any concerns should be discussed directly with your physician or specialist before you decide to cancel your appointment."

January 19

Today is the last day of Trump. We will be glad to see the backside of him. I really enjoyed the meme of them carting him out of his office still seated in his desk chair mumbling about the election.

I attended the Operations meeting. They are trying to navigate the constant changes in policy. Both the President of the hospital and the coordinator of the COHT are working, under order by the province, at one of the LTC homes. The home had a severe Covid-19 outbreak resulting in many deaths of residents and staff.

January 21

I spent one and half hours on the COHT call. There is too much happening and too few staff to deal with it all. I could feel the stress through the internet cable.

I arranged to speak to the President of Information Orillia, who manages the Seniors News Line, about him joining the COHT.

I confirmed that the patient volunteer will speak to the Chair of the JET next Wednesday to discuss her family's devastating experience with the current health care system.

January 22

I spoke with the President of Information Orillia. He agreed to attend the next COHT meeting and will decide after he gets a better understanding of the committee's mandate. I sent an email to the Coordinator of the COHT and instructed him to send an invitation.

January 23

I sent a signed attestation to mom's home. The attestation confirmed that I had completed my PPE training. In addition to weekly Covid-19 tests, I will need to be retrained and sign an attestation every month.

Health Canada approved a rapid Covid-19 test for emergency use. The company Spartan Bioscience had previously recalled the test last spring over concerns expressed by Health Canada. My understanding is that the test has a problem with false positives. False positives will cause problems with staffing, case number tracking, and increased cost and time for repeat testing.

January 24

I prepared the news summary for tomorrow's recording. There was so much important news, including the highly contagious and deadly UK variant of Covid-19 detected in Barrie and deaths in LTC homes, that I exceeded my normal time.

January 25

I prepared and recorded my news update.

"Ontario reported 2417 new Covid-19 cases today.

The province reported 50 deaths today, 25 were residents of long-term care homes.

On Friday, the Simcoe Muskoka District Health Unit reported 112 new cases of Covid-19 in the region.

There is also evidence of a Covid-19 variant strain that is much more contagious and deadly. There are 37 people from Simcoe County hospitalized with Covid-19.

There have been 14,583 doses of the Pfizer-BioNTech vaccine against Covid-19 administered in Simcoe Muskoka to health care workers in local hospitals, long-term care and retirement homes, as well as to all eligible long-term care home residents. No doses were administered yesterday.

The health unit reports 927 individuals from the region have received both doses of the vaccine.

Due to a shortage in vaccine supply, the health unit is reorganizing its vaccine rollout with a priority of getting at least one dose to retirement home residents, all eligible long-term care residents have received their first dose. It's unclear if the health unit will be able to provide a second dose within the twenty-one-day time frame to all those who received their first dose of the vaccine.

The Ontario government has declared a state of emergency, the second since the start of the pandemic, and a stay at-home order is in effect until at least February 11, 2021.

“The presence of the United Kingdom variant of Covid-19 at a long-term care home in Barrie could mean more changes to protective measures in long-term care homes, the local community, and abroad,” said Dr. Charles Gardner, the medical officer of health for the Simcoe Muskoka District Health Unit.

On Saturday, public health officials confirmed the more virulent UK variant is present at the LTC home, where the death toll has now reached thirty-two.

There are 127 residents — which represents all but two residents — who have tested positive for the virus, as well as 84 workers, which represents approximately half of the entire staff. Six residents and one staff member are currently hospitalized at Royal Victoria Regional Health Centre (RVH).

The outbreak at the 137-bed long-term care home was first declared on January 8.

This week, it was reported that a worker may have brought the virus into the Barrie facility after being in contact with an international traveller. Gardner was asked if charges could be laid if someone wasn't following quarantine rules.

"When we looked at the situation, we actually did not see violation of any of the recommendations from the province, nor was there a violation of the Quarantine Act with regards to the individual who was travelling," he said during a weekend Zoom call with reporters. "So, the exposure in question did not take place out in the community."

The staff member who contracted the virus did not show symptoms at the beginning when they went to work, the doctor noted.

"They were asymptomatic when they were tested routinely," Gardner said.

Public health officials have been reluctant to release any information that could identify either the staff member or the traveller, but Gardner did confirm the traveller is a resident of Simcoe-Muskoka.

"There's no requirement to be in isolation and not go into work solely because one has been in contact with a traveller who's asymptomatic," Gardner said.

"We need to keep learning about this virus as we go," he added. "I have no doubt that, with this variant, we're going to continue to have to change and tighten up requirements."

Questions have also been raised about staff at the LTC home going between rooms of residents who were positive for the virus and others who were not.

"I would agree that the home never successfully put in place the kind of cohorting - where you maintain the restriction on the movement of staff, or the exposure of staff to cases and non-cases," Gardner said.

"That was something that certainly was not the optimum practice in an outbreak and that wasn't established, in part because of how quickly this spread and in part because the number of staff that became ill, they had such a difficulty maintaining the adequate staffing in the first place."

Cohorting is a strategy to reduce risk of transmission by assigning health-care workers to patients or groups of patients based on patient exposure or infection.

Gardner said it can be "challenging" to do that, however, during a fast-moving outbreak.

"This moved very quickly," he said. "There were forty cases that emerged over the course of a single weekend at the very beginning. The rapid pace made it difficult to put those measures in place."

The President of the company which operates the home, said the virus came into the long-term care home so quickly they couldn't achieve cohorting "in a quick and timely fashion."

With so many staff and team members infected at the home, Gardner said they have had to take a multi-faceted approach to ensure staffing levels are sufficient at the facility. The company has reallocated staff and also brought in temporary workers from outside organizations, such as the Red Cross.

An occupational health and safety team has been formed involving the health unit and other health-care partners. They also want to make sure all employees are offered the vaccine, Gardner said.

"From what we have seen, the uptake for this has been very, very strong, but we need to continue that as new people come into the facility," he added.

There will be ongoing monitoring at the home through rapid testing by Orillia Soldiers' Memorial Hospital (OSMH), which has been granted temporary leadership of the long-term care home following an order under the Health Protection and Promotion Act (HPPA).

Testing will be done on a twice-weekly basis. Anyone who shows symptoms or who has a positive result will be placed in isolation at home, or hospitalized if needed.

Gardner said they hope to contain the variant to the site and limit spread into the community. This includes "a stricter threshold" for people who are at higher risk and more intensive follow-up. In cases where the person cannot isolate at home, they could be put up in a hotel to reduce the risk of spread to household members, he added.

"Our goal is to avoid transmission into the community," the doctor said.

Gardner conceded community spread involving the UK variant is likely already happening.

"It's certainly on the edge," he said. "It would depend on their contacts beyond their household and whether or not we're starting to see spread there. We haven't seen that yet, but we're on the very edge."

Gardner said health officials also want to protect long-term care homes and retirement facilities from community spread.

If outbreaks are seen at other facilities, Gardner said he will have the genome sequencing done to determine whether the variant is showing up in those other facilities.

With the local emergence of the UK variant, Gardner was asked if any modifications to protocols or protective measures will be put in place at other long-term care homes in Simcoe-Muskoka.

About the home with the outbreak, case and contact management has already changed to identify people who are considered high-risk.

"If in fact there's been an exposure that's just momentary, rather than fifteen minutes or more, we're considering that a high-risk contact and those individuals go into isolation or quarantine," Gardner said.

As well, people in full protective gear who have been in a confined space for more than thirty minutes with an infected person, they will also be considered a high-risk exposure. The isolation period for such instances is being extended from ten days to fourteen.

"The experience that has been seen with the UK variant in other countries has been of a higher viral load and therefore possibly a longer period of viral shedding," said Gardner, "resulting in a longer period of isolation. We certainly will have to learn from this with regard to what we do at other sites. The whole province will have to learn as we go."

"All eyes are watching us right now," the doctor added.

Gardner said the situation at the home will have a "profound" effect on other long-term care homes.

"We all need to be on the alert," he said.

The immunization of all residents' retirement homes is another immediate change in protocol at long-term care homes, Gardner said. Last weekend, vaccinations were completed for all residents of long-term care homes in Simcoe-Muskoka. That focus has now shifted to retirement homes in the region. There are still 16 homes to go, which Gardner expected to be done by Wednesday."

This news segment alerted me to the fact the health agencies seem to be flying by the seat of their pants. I do not understand why they are not following the Pandemic Influenza Plan developed in 2004 after the successful management of the SARS pandemic in 2003. The core goals of the plan were to prioritize saving lives through infection prevention, accelerated vaccine production using the influenza production and formulation methods, and treatment access while navigating essential services.

The residents at mom's home received their first dose of Moderna vaccine today. I called to remind them that mom cannot receive it due to her autoimmune disorders.

January 26

I called a friend and discussed her son's condition. He is a fifty-year-old with mental and physical challenges since birth. All adult day care homes have closed their doors indefinitely and the government has cancelled their funding. I told her that staying home may be the safest thing for them. The problem will be after the pandemic, because she will have difficulty managing on her own.

January 28

I have an appointment this morning for my Covid-19 test and I dread going. Sometimes it feels like that are poking the swab into my brain and last time there was blood when I blew my nose.

January 29

The meeting with the JET and the patient was at 4:30 pm. We had a frank discussion and agreed that follow up is required. I volunteered to organize the discussions.

Chapter 13 – FEBRUARY 2021

February 1

I recorded the news update.

“Dozens of city employees went on strike this past Saturday.

In a news release issued Thursday evening, the City of Orillia noted that unionized staff in the Environment and Infrastructure Services Group will be on strike.

They include staff from water/wastewater, waste diversion, operations (including roads and winter maintenance), environmental officers, and electricians.

Fifty-eight staff are included in the collective bargaining unit.

The city says it has a contingency plan “to maintain all critical services to the public, which includes bringing in outside contractors and redeploying city staff.

The strike will not impact drinking water and wastewater treatment. The city’s Waste Diversion Site will remain open and garbage collection will not be affected. Winter maintenance will be carried out in accordance with provincial minimum maintenance standards and road maintenance will continue.

Temporary Pfizer vaccine delays are largely behind us.

Pfizer had scaled back its delivery schedule last month as the pharmaceutical company upgraded its manufacturing plant in Belgium to boost production of its vaccine.

Federal Procurement Minister Anita Anand says Canadians can soon expect the country's Covid-19 inoculation campaign to pick up steam after Canada's vaccine rollout was temporarily beset by delivery delays and reduced shipments of doses. They recently received assurances from the vaccine manufacturers that those delays were temporary. From February 15 onwards, vaccine rollout will take on a steep incline. Many health care workers and residents of long-term care and retirement homes are scheduled to receive their second dose. The Couchiching Ontario Health Team is preparing for the receipt and administration of Covid-19 vaccine to the public as soon as it is available."

The article about the Pfizer manufacturing plant concerned me. When a manufacturing plant for a biological product is upgraded, it usually means changes in the manufacturing process. Typically, the changes can affect the quality of the final product, requiring safety and effectiveness to be re-established in clinical trials. It appears that they were exempt from that requirement. This means that the smaller batches used in the original clinical trial were different than the batches that will be administered to the masses and that the safety and effectiveness of the vaccine can no longer be assumed.

February 4

I went for my Covid-19 test and then participated in a hospital Operations meeting. The meeting focused on staff Covid-19 infections, vaccination, staff capacity, LTC home outbreaks, ICU capacity, PPE shortages and restart of surgeries when PPE supplies are stable.

Case numbers and the variant cases are declining. Staff have only received their first dose. LTC residents will be given their second dose by February 9.

I pointed out that it is interesting that case numbers and deaths are declining significantly even though very few people have received the vaccine. Hopefully, the vaccine will not be required to end the pandemic as Trudeau claimed.

The organizer of the Senior News Line contacted me to discuss advertising. She believes that there are more people who can benefit from the health news updates I am providing.

February 11

I participated in a video call with the Senior News Line team of volunteers. The meeting went well and we came up with a few ideas to spread the word further. It was nice to see the faces of the other news readers. I was told that the health news I provided on Mondays was the most popular according to the call statistics and a survey of users.

February 12

I chaired the Northern Patient Family Advisory Network meeting and there was much discussion about the latest lockdowns, the co-variant, and hospital visits.

February 15

I recorded the news:

“I hope you enjoyed Valentine’s Day. If you missed it, grab your phone and call someone you care about.

The Province's reopening plan could create 'confusion,'

If Covid-19 infection rates trend positively, non-essential stores could reopen doors to limited capacity by February 16.

But don't expect unfettered and unrestricted access to your favourite big box store anytime soon.

No in-person shopping at non-essential retailers is permitted in regions where the stay-at-home order remains in effect, which is most of the province.

Non-essential retailers will be permitted to open their doors at a patron capacity of twenty-five per cent. This applies to retailers like hardware and liquor stores, discount and big box stores. Retailers must have a screening system in place for patrons.

Retail businesses will welcome their ability to reopen under restricted capacity. The business community will continue to prove their commitment to safety protocols to protect their workers and customers to keep their doors open."

February 17

One of the doctors from the hospital called to ask me to go to the Rotary Place for a walk through of the Covid-19 Vaccination Clinic. I made several suggestions for improvement based on my years of clinical trial experience. I also asked to review the Consent Form that patients will read and sign to ensure that they are aware of the potential risks. I said that Informed Consent is a requirement for all experimental products. I was told that there was no consent form because the government does not consider the vaccines to be experimental and stated that the emergency regulations exempt signed consent. This raised alarm bells for me. How could the government allow an experimental product, which the Covid-19 vaccine clearly is, to be administered to healthy individuals without informing them that the product has not been fully tested and that the long-term safety and effectiveness of the product is unknown? This does not provide the information required to perform a risk versus benefit analysis by their physician. No one seemed to be interested in my concerns, and I left the clinic frustrated.

I received an invitation to attend a meeting of the PFAC Chairs next week. I sent a draft Term of Reference for the PFAC to the JET and a request we share it with the PFAN.

February 18

I have a busy day ahead of me.

Covid-19 test at 11:30 am,

COHT meeting at 1:30 pm, and

PFAC meeting at 2:30 pm.

I sent out emails to the Senior News Line Team with copies of the draft posters and requests that they print and distribute them.

February 22

I recorded the news.

"Roberta Place residents and workers were recognized with a special drive-by parade.

Staff from North Simcoe Muskoka Specialized Geriatrics Services were joined by local partners and Barrie firefighters to show their support for people living and working at Roberta Place. Several staff of the hospital were deployed to the long-term care facility for several weeks to assist with the management of the Covid-19 outbreak.

The outbreak was declared on January 8. In just over a month, there were 67confirmed resident deaths linked to the virus, three more considered probables, and one death of an essential caregiver.

The outbreak was declared over on February 18.

All long-term care and retirement home residents in Orillia who wanted Covid-19 vaccine have received their second dose. They will not be fully protected for another couple of weeks.

The Chippewas of Rama First Nations moved into the red zone on February 16 and have been offered Covid-19 vaccine.

The Couchiching Ontario Health Team are now gearing up at the Rotary Place to offer vaccine to seniors over eighty years old by appointment only. Contact your primary care provider and stayed tuned for more information.

When you have received your Covid-19 vaccine, please continue to practice safety measures to prevent spread in our community.

If you are enjoying the Orillia Seniors News Line please share with your family, friends and neighbours who do not have access to the internet.

One of the patient advisors called to discuss concerns about cancer care, screening, elective surgeries, wait times, communication and end of life visits. I promised to forward these concerns to the hospital Operations Committee meeting tomorrow.

February 23

I spent two hours working on PFAN documents and strategy.

I spent thirty minutes with the Operations Committee. I raised the concerns received by the patient advisor yesterday.

February 24

At the meeting of the regional OHT PFAC we discussed compensation for the PFAC members. I suggested that rather than a stipend, members be reimbursed for expenses, such as travel. This would signal the importance of their work and there was unanimous agreement.

After the meeting, I revised the COHT PFAC Terms of Reference to include reimbursement and sent it to the JET for review. If there is agreement, a budget would be required.

I received a call from the LHIN. They offered a bed for mom at one of my preferred LTC homes. I expressed my concern about the outbreaks in LTC homes in Ontario and that I would prefer to delay mom's transfer until the risk is over. She said that she understood and agreed. She recommended that I speak to mom's current facility before the LHIN takes any action. After the call, I spoke to my mom's home, and they assured me that they will continue to care for her until after the pandemic. I called the LHIN and they agreed to remove mom from the crisis list. I was told that due to the unusual circumstances of the pandemic, she will remain on the waiting list, and I can change the priority at any time. Normally, if you refuse a bed, you are taken off the waiting list, and a new application would be required.

February 26

The elderly neighbour across the street called. Both her and her husband are in their late eighties. The earliest appointment they could get for a Covid-19 vaccine is in June. I sent an email to the street neighbours advising them to make an appointment as soon as possible.

Chapter 14 - MARCH 2021

March 1

I recorded the news.

"A Covid-19 vaccination clinic has been established at the Rotary Place. It opens Wednesday March 3.

If you are eighty-five or older you can book your appointment NOW online on the SIMCOE MUSKOKA DISTRICT HEALTH UNIT website.

If you are unable to book your appointment online call someone you know to do it for you. There is a number to call to book, but it is almost impossible to get through.

They will be accepting bookings, one week at a time. The number of appointments is based on the number of doses of vaccine available each week.

If you do not see any available slots add your name to the wait list. They will contact you with a date and time when available.

Any adults on chronic home care service will also be included in this phase.

Following the 85-plus cohort, those 80 to 85 will be getting vaccinated as of March 15,

75 to 79 - April 15,

70 to 74 - May 1, and

65 to 69 - June 1.

These dates are contingent upon consistent vaccine and PPE supplies.

Today, the Simcoe Muskoka area goes back into lockdown.

These decisions are not made lightly and consider many factors. This time smaller retail stores may stay open with reduced capacity of twenty-five percent and larger stores of fifty percent. It can be done safely if everyone wears their masks and try to limit the time spent in each store.

The reason Simcoe Muskoka has moved into Lockdown is we have the largest number of UK variant cases in Ontario. The variant is more contagious than the original strain, and results in more severe disease. Moving into Lockdown may help stop a third wave or limit its severity.

During the pandemic, the Couchiching Ontario Health Team has been working diligently to improve health care services for fragile seniors in our area. This team is a partnership of organizations with a shared purpose, shared resources, improved communication and coordination.

In addition to Soldiers Hospital and the Couchiching Family Health

Team, other members include the Sharing Place, Lighthouse, Helping Hands, Paramedic services, Home and Community Care, Public Health, Palliative Care Networks.

A network of patient, family and caregiver advisors is currently under development to support the Health Team. More information will be available in the coming weeks.

The JET meeting lasted from noon to 2:00 pm. We focused on the staffing, PPE and vaccine supply issues, the vaccination clinic, and the drop in the number of Covid-19 cases. The government is putting pressure to resume non-urgent surgeries and procedures. This should be good news, but the hospital is anxious about supplies. We also discussed the PFAC Terms of Reference and the restart of member recruitment. There is only one member – me. I said that the JET needs to take responsibility and begin the process of bringing on new members.

March 2

I spoke to a potential co-chair of the PFAC. I promised to send her the Terms of Reference and a membership application form. We will arrange an interview with members of the JET.

I also spoke to another person who may be interested in becoming a member of the PFAC. I will send her the Terms of Reference and an application form.

I spoke to the Chair of the hospital Ethics Committee and then sent a confirmation email. I told her that due to my heavy workload as a volunteer and the care of my mother, I must resign from the Ethics Committee.

Truth be told, I do not agree with the policies and procedures dictated by the government. The triage of patients is especially stressful. I am not convinced that the use of ventilators is safe for patients with inflamed lungs. Ventilators force oxygen into the lungs and if the lungs are clogged, severe damage may be caused. I asked why they did not use cytokines to reduce the lung inflammation. I was told that the government would not approve anti-inflammatory drugs for treatment of Covid-19. I also asked why they did not use ivermectin or hydroxychloroquine when patients demanded them. The same answer was given. The government will not approve their use for treatment of Covid-19 and hospitals cannot legally use any drug that has not been approved by the regulators.

I do not understand the difference between the approval of experimental vaccines with unknown safety and effectiveness profiles and the experimental use of safe treatments that may prevent deaths. My concerns about the limited options for patients and my suspicions about the motives to support only Covid-19 vaccines, made my participation in triage exercises extremely difficult.

March 3

The Orillia Covid-19 Vaccination Clinic opened today. I checked and there is no Informed Consent being used. This means that the recipients are not aware of the potential risks or the groups not recommended to receive the vaccine, for example pregnant women.

March 4

I went for my Covid-19 test and I could see the vaccination clinic on the other side of the building. As I recommended, they designated separate entrances for testing and vaccination.

As suggested by the JET, I chatted with the Chair of the PFAC for the Penetang Correction Center. She is willing to provide guidance in developing the COHT PFAC, help with interviews and orientation of new members. She is not willing to be a member of the COHT PFAC.

I discussed the PFAC with three other possible new members. During the discussion, the following questions were raised:

Who approves the PFAC members?

What is the minimum number of members before we restart the PFAC?

What are the qualifications of the members?

How often are the meetings held? They need to be held at night and by video call to accommodate members who work in the day.

Will they be provided compensation?

Two of the people indicated interest. The third was not interested in a long-term commitment. All those I spoke to were concerned that the advisory committee is just for show and that we will not make any positive impact on the system. They felt that the government was just paying lip service to the public by establishing these "so-called" advisory committees. I did my best to convince them that our involvement is necessary to ensure a better outcome.

The secretary of the Ethics Committee brought me a gift and card. It was such a nice gesture. We chatted in the driveway about the strain on the hospital staff over the past year. She said that several of the members agree with me but will not speak up. They are all employed by the hospital and fear for their jobs. They were disappointed that I will not continue to be an advocate for the patients on the Ethics Committee. I said that I am still an advocate on the Patient and Family Advisory Committee.

I sent an email to the JET coordinator listing the questions from the PFAC candidates. To keep the process moving, I will need to get back to the candidates with the answers as soon as possible.

March 7

I worked on the PFAN Terms of Reference and sent a draft to the Network.

March 8

A neighbour down the street called to discuss getting the vaccine. Her husband has an autoimmune condition and is over eighty. I told her to discuss the risks and benefits with her physician. If they decide to proceed, I will help them make an appointment online. I sent her a copy of the vaccine information brochure I obtained from the vaccination clinic. I told her to give it to their doctor.

March 10

I spoke to the PFAC coordinator and hashed out the Terms of Reference, Application form, interview process and reimbursement. We also discussed the comments from the patients and caregivers I already interviewed. He will put the items on the next JET meeting agenda.

March 12

Mom's home changed the visitation rules once again. Covid-19 testing and PPE training are now required every two weeks. I can only visit mom from 1:00 to 4:00 pm on Tuesdays, Thursdays and Sundays. This is not good. She is barely benefitting from daily visits, and she is always worse on Thursdays and Fridays because I have not been allowed to visit on Wednesdays. I fear that her condition will further deteriorate with only three weekly visits. There is nothing I can do because the home is private. I cannot wait until I can move her into a different facility.

I spoke to my friend with the mentally challenged son. He is not doing well and misses the stimulation received at adult daycare. The Ontario government closed all adult daycare facilities and do not intend to reopen them in the future. There is so much evidence that the healthcare system is broken in so many ways.

March 13

I called mom's home about the changes to their visitor rules. I sent an email questioning the rationale, as it appears to be based on convenience for the staff and not about the benefits for the residents.

One of the hospital volunteers called about the Senior News Line pamphlets. She will distribute them to the Common Roof, a place for vulnerable people.

March 14

I recorded my health news summary.

"The Rotary Place opened its vaccination clinic on March 3.

The facility houses both the Covid-19 assessment center and the vaccination clinic, which are accessed by the doors on east side of the building.

A family member or friend can book your on-line appointment if you are unable to do so yourself. You can also be put on a wait list.

Or you can call the Simcoe Muskoka District Health for assistance in booking an appointment.

Alert: When the clinic calls those on the wait list to book an appointment, they never ask for your social insurance number or banking information. Do not give out this information under any circumstances. They will only ask you to confirm your date of birth.

When you go for your vaccination, arrive precisely the time of your appointment. Registration and vaccination will take five to ten minutes. You will be monitored for fifteen to thirty minutes before you may leave.

Lately in the news there have been claims of serious adverse reactions. Health Canada claims that these are extremely rare and that they are closely monitoring the reports for any trends.

Health Canada has now approved a total of five Covid-19 vaccines from four different companies. Hopefully, the new vaccines will increase the number of doses available, and this will increase the number of appointments each week.

Daily rapid testing serves as early warning of potential Covid-19 infection at Long Term Care facilities

Since results from the antigen test do not require lab processing and are available in thirty minutes, long term care homes can move faster at the first potential signs of infection.

Prior to the rapid antigen testing, weekly PCR testing was used. Now, testing of staff is performed daily.

The new testing program started at all four county-operated long-term care homes last week.

I felt like a hypocrite presenting the vaccine information as dictated to me by the medical community. It is not appropriate for me to provide my opinions about the information. If I did so, I would be removed from the news line program. I need to keep providing the crucial information using this vehicle and find other ways to warn people about the risks.

I visited mom and when I was ready to leave, I chatted with one of the PSWs. She is not happy with the changes. She agreed that frequent visits by the essential caregivers benefits the residents and provides some relief for the PSW staff. The home seemed to be concerned that people visiting at all hours, meant that they needed to keep the rooms and residents in good condition all the time. By limiting the number of days and times, they could reduce their services, and no one would notice.

I sent an update to the neighbours about the vaccine and the Senior News Line. In my update, I also included the warnings provided in the vaccine information sheet and a suggestion that they speak to their physician about the risks.

March 16

I visited mom in the afternoon. She was in bed still in her night gown. Her breakfast and lunch were on the dresser. She had nothing to eat or drink today. I fed her and got some juice and tea into her. I spoke to the supervisor about it and told her that I am very upset.

When I arrived home, I called the LHIN and put mom back on the crisis list.

I scheduled a Zoom call with one of the councillors of the Rama Reservation to discuss a meeting with their council and their Health Officer about Rama members joining the Patient and Caregiver Advisory Committee to the COHT. This meeting was approved by the JET.

March 17

I had a great discussion with the Rama councillor. I sent him the Terms of Reference for the PFAC and he agreed to set up the video call with the council. I asked the coordinator of the Senior News Line to also send information to him about the online service.

I sent a copy of the poster for the Senior News Line to the Volunteer Supervisor at the hospital. She promised to put copies at the front entrance.

I am now working with the Secretary of the COHT to distribute PFAC meeting minutes. She will attend all meetings, draft the minutes and send them to me for review and approval before sharing them.

March 18

As recommended by the RAMA Councillor, I organized a video call with the head of Barrie Area Native Advisory Circle (BANAC) to discuss the PFAC.

March 22

Our elderly next-door neighbour called to ask about the vaccine for him and his wife. He also wants help booking their appointments online which he found very difficult to navigate. I gave him my Coles notes about the risks and left it to him to decide. He said that he would think about it.

March 23

Our son called to discuss the new Covid-19 vaccines, specifically the mRNA products produced by Pfizer and Moderna. He asked if they would modify the body's DNA. I explained that the platform is mRNA and will not have the ability to change DNA. I also explained that only a very small amount is administered in the muscle and therefore, it would not likely travel to other parts of the body.

However, there is a concern that in rare cases the vaccine may be injected into a vein and therefore the entire body would be exposed to the mRNA and spike protein. There are no data about how long the mRNA would remain in the body. For as long as it is in the body it would continue to produce the spike protein. I described it as a small spike protein manufacturing plant.

They are considering getting the vaccine if, and when, it is available for his forty-year-old age group. I told him that I will continue to research it further and we can discuss it again when it becomes available.

March 27

Our car and RV license stickers arrived by mail. One good thing is that during the pandemic, the fees were waived by the government.

March 30

As recommended by the JET, I met with the Chair of the PFAC for Way Point to discuss assistance with the PFAC member recruitment. She is paid staff and cannot help me. She suggested that I speak to one of the Patient members of their regional Ontario Health Team and provided her contact information. I sent her an email requesting a video call.

March 31

The Federal government announced that Connaught is receiving funding to build a new vaccine manufacturing plant. It is interesting that Connaught did not develop a Covid-19 vaccine or mRNA vaccine. They probably knew that it was not possible to do it properly in the required timeframe. I am so happy that the company who employed me for the first twenty years of my career, continues to put safety before profit.

Chapter 15 – APRIL 2021

April 5

I expected to have a video call at 2:00 pm with one of the representatives of BANAC to discuss PFAC membership and Indigenous representation. It was booked a while ago and I sent reminders. I waited for thirty minutes, and no one joined me.

April 6

I spoke to the representative of the Regional OHT about assistance with our PFAC recruitment and orientation. We will work together to prepare a plan and guidelines for approval by the JET.

I organized a call to speak to the COHT coordinator tomorrow about the failed call with the BANAC representative.

April 7

I managed to reach the individual from BANAC. She apologized for the mix up with the meeting. She agreed to spend some time with me now and we had an excellent discussion –

She said that we need to separate engagement from patient input.

We will need to create a separate safe council for indigenous patients.

The COHT needs to add Indigenous Engagement at a high level.

The BANAC has worked with the LHIN since 2006, and they hope that they will not be starting from scratch with the COHT. She provided the name and contact information of the LHIN liaison.

She explained that the Indigenous Health Circle, which includes RAMA, is not part of BANAC.

She agreed to discuss a PFAC Indigenous Working Group with the leaders of BANAC and then get back to me.

It is all very complicated and confusing. I followed-up with a call to the COHT coordinator to provide an update. I also raised several other pressing issues –

My discussions with the representatives of Waypoint and the Regional OHT.

The provincial government had just announced the postponement of the LHIN dissolution and did not set a date for it to occur. The Liberal government formed the LHIN. When the Conservatives took over, they planned to replace the LHIN with Ontario Health Teams. We now have two groups managing similar things. What are we doing to ensure there are no overlaps or things slipping between the cracks?

I also raised the concern that if the Conservatives do not win the upcoming election, the Ontario Health Teams and the Health Care System may be negatively impacted.

We agreed that I would summarize my discussion with BANAC and the issues I raised about the LHIN and the upcoming election and present it during the JET meeting on Monday. I will distribute a summary document to the members over the weekend.

April 10

I chatted with a couple who have been our friends for over forty years. It was not a great discussion. They are both very depressed. He needs home care, but it is hard to get right now. They spoke to CCAC (that is the former acronym for the LHIN) and they have been put on a waiting list. They cannot get out to get the Covid-19 vaccine, and they inquired about someone coming to their home. It is not possible due to the complicated storage requirements. I tried to convince them that if they stay home and do not expose themselves to others, they should be safe. They can get whatever they need delivered to their door.

April 12

I recorded the health news.

"The stay-at-home order for all of Ontario is still in effect.

The Covid-19 numbers are rising. On Sunday, the province reported 4,456 new cases and 21 deaths. Most cases are Covid-19 variants. These increases have delayed surgeries and cancer treatments because hospitals are over capacity. A new ruling in the province allows patients to be transferred to another hospital even if they do not give their consent. This will impact both Barry and Orillia hospitals who will receive patients transferred from the Greater Toronto Area.

How do you know if your Covid-19 appointment booking was successful? Look for the screen with the Ontario logo at the top and the blue check mark!

IMPORTANT: When booking on the provincial booking system, you must book dose one and dose two appointments for the booking to be successful. If you only choose an appointment for dose one and exit, your booking has NOT been completed.

With a successful booking you will receive an email confirmation immediately.

You will need to bring the confirmation to your appointment.

A new Virtual Assistant has been launched to help with Covid-19 case management. It is a new text messaging tool which will increase the speed and volume of case management.

If you recently tested positive for Covid-19, you may receive a text message from the health unit asking you to complete a secure personal assessment form online. This will allow you to share information about your health status, the people you have been in close contact with, and other essential information to help with contact tracing and follow-up.

After you submit your information, you may receive a phone call from a provincial public health partner to collect further information.

The form is voluntary and will take approximately ten minutes to complete. You can opt out by texting the word STOP."

I attended the JET meeting where we discussed the update that I provided. They agreed to accept the offer of assistance from the Regional OHT. I will follow up with their representative.

April 15

The COHT meeting went well. I provided the PFAC updates and after the meeting, the RAMA councillor sent me an email to let me know that the RAMA council will discuss possible ways to get involved with PFAC.

April 19

I recorded the news.

As a result of the rapid increase in transmission rates of Covid-19 and its variants, the province announced new strengthening measures that include extending the emergency declaration to May 20, implementing new restrictions and enhancing enforcement.

The new restrictions will apply province-wide:

Outdoor gatherings will be strictly limited to members of the same household, only, or with one other household if those individuals live alone.

In-person shopping at stores that primarily sell food and pharmaceutical goods will be restricted to twenty-five percent occupancy.

All non-essential workplaces in the construction sector will be closed (e.g., shopping malls, hotels and office towers).

All outdoor amenities will be closed (e.g. soccer fields, basketball courts and other multi-use fields).

Garage and yard sales are prohibited.

Moving into these enhanced restrictions includes a number of closures and restrictions for Ramara township's municipal services that will begin on Monday, April 19. These include:

Closure of the Township Administration Building and all buildings to the public.

Ramara Public Library will continue to be closed to the public and offer virtual programming and curbside pickup.

Ramara Recreation department will continue to provide all virtual programing, but all curbside programming is cancelled.

The building and planning department will continue to accept all residential applications electronically or by hard copy dropped off in the outside drop box.

All non-residential building permit applications will be examined on a case-by-case basis, so please call the building department prior to submission.

All building inspections will continue on Tuesdays and Thursdays.

Short-Term Rental Accommodations are strictly prohibited, unless it is rented to a person in need.

Those in highest risk health category plus one essential caregiver may now book a Covid-19 vaccine appointment.

These include:

Organ or stem cell transplant

Neurological disease, such as MS, in which respiratory function may be compromised (Side note: MS is an autoimmune disorder. According to the manufacturer's information, the vaccine should not be administered to those with autoimmune conditions).

Hematological malignance diagnosed within the past year

Severe Kidney disease.

While camping is not permitted under the current provincial shutdown restrictions, parks and heritage sites across Ontario and Canada are accepting reservations for later in the season.

The regular season for camping in most parks typically doesn't start until May. With stay-at-home orders extended until May 20, it will be later this year.

Due to the nature of shared and common spaces at campgrounds, visitors must complete any requirements for self-isolation before arriving.

Visitors are also asked to arrive prepared to be self-sufficient with extra hygiene supplies, food and their own water.

I had a very informative and constructive meeting with the Medical Director of the Rama Health Portfolio. She is also a member of the BANAC Indigenous Health Circle. If the head of BANAC agrees to sit on the PFAC, she could bring the patients' voices to the table. Those indigenous members who do not live on the Rama reservation use most of the community services, including the local food bank. I will let her know what BANAC has to say. She added that if the BANAC Health Circle joins the PFAC, Rama would not create a separate committee. They would be represented via the Health Circle.

April 22

Today I chaired the first meeting of the COHT PFAC. We covered a lot in one hour and it was agreed that we will meet every two weeks. The following topics were discussed.

We reviewed and discussed the GAP analysis and COHT Shared

Purpose and Guiding Principles.

The budget for the next year has been established.

Human resources for PFAC support have been identified.

PFAC decision-making power has been determined. The Chair of PFAC is a voting member of the Joint Executive Team for the COHT.

We are in the process of determining the ideal number of members, qualifications, representation and questions before interviewing.

Members will determine the vision of this committee.

We need to finalize the recruitment and selection process.

How will we know that this group has impacted the work of the OHT? What are the things we can do up front to make sure we have that in place?

The current challenge is how we can improve specific agencies from a patient & family perspective within the OHT. How do we work with so many agencies?

I provided an updated Engagement with Rama First Nations.

I spoke with the Executive Director of Rama Health Portfolio and with a member of BANAC. RAMA is not a member of BANAC, they are a member of the Indigenous Health Circle of BANAC. BANAC has been working with the LIHN, and they are not sure who they will work with when the LIHN dissolves. It was agreed during the Rama discussion, that if the BANAC Indigenous Health Circle puts a member on our PFAC they will bring the voices of the patients of the indigenous community, including Rama, to the PFAC. We will need to determine the implications of a non-patient PFAC member. The JET agreed that I will continue the discussions with Rama and BANAC.

I went for my Covid-19 test this morning and there was a long line-up for the vaccine and no line-up for the test.

April 23

I sent the PFAC minutes to the COHT secretary for distribution to the JET members.

April 26

I recorded the health news.

“The third Covid-19 wave was explained by the Simcoe County Health:

The Covid-19 pandemic started a year ago. When it started there was the extreme fear of the unknown. We didn’t know how bad the pandemic would be. The local medical community worried that we would have huge surges of Covid-19 patients in our area and that they would overwhelm hospitals’ critical care.

The first and second waves came and we in Orillia did not have the surges in Covid-19 patients we expected. However, in Covid-19 hot spots like the Greater Toronto Area, where they had overwhelmed ER's and overflowing ICU's during the second wave, the sacrifices made during the first two waves appeared to help stem the flood of Covid-19 infections.

This third wave is different. This third wave has variants that are more contagious and cause more serious disease in the younger population.

When a patient gets admitted to the ICU or hospital their family can't visit them. They are left with speaking to them on the phone or seeing them on their iPads or tablets. Their "new" family is their healthcare team, who will take care of them twenty-four hours a day and seven days a week.

Why is the situation so dire right now?

Ontario currently has 1846 FULL ICU beds. There are approximately 700 hundred patients with Covid-19 in ICUs across the province. The rest of the ICU beds are filled with patients that have had heart attacks, strokes, motor vehicle accidents etc... In Simcoe County, our local ICUs are full, and our hospitals have accepted dozens of transfers from the Greater Toronto Area hospitals because they are bursting at the seams.

What can you do?

Be Safe

When away from home and in-doors always wear your mask.

Consider wearing a double mask (preferably medical 3-layer mask) for extra protection against the more contagious variants.

Reduce your chance of ending up in hospital.

Try to avoid doing any risky activities that could lead to hospitalization. If you choose to do a risky activity, be extra, extra careful. In the ER in cottage country, we see at least one trauma a week which must be flown via ORNGE helicopter to a trauma hospital in Toronto. When you see the orange ORNGE helicopter that is most likely a trauma victim or a critically ill patient. What are the causes of trauma in cottage country? ATV, jet skiing, boating, and motorcycle accidents are very common. If you are operating a chainsaw or climbing a ladder, do it safely.

Socialization is important for seniors and youth alike but now is not the time to get together in person.

We all have the responsibility to be safe.

Ontario has now banned outdoor gatherings with anyone outside of your household. When this stay-at-home order is finished, if you are going to get together with someone, please do it outside. Transmission outside is less likely, but still theoretically possible. Consider wearing a mask if you can't maintain six feet of distance or if you are down wind. Meeting indoors is risky, especially if it is for more than fifteen minutes. "

April 28

I was interviewed by a member of Health Ontario about the COHT, its mission, framework, budget and patient involvement. I commented that although we have established a PFAC, it is in name only and there has been very little patient and caregiver input. I alone cannot represent all patients and caregivers. I said that we are in the process of finalizing the PFAC.

I learned today that the province is opening the door to redeploying staff within hospitals to address the most critical needs. The staff shortages in critical care have been the result of sick leave, quarantine due to Covid-19 exposure and retirement. The hospitals will review the most recent directive with their union partners to gain a better understanding of where available skills may be a match for the required work, with the understanding that team members are only assigned tasks or asked to deliver services that they are reasonably qualified to provide.

April 30

I sent an email to all my committees letting them know that I will be away for a couple of weeks and may not be available to attend the meetings by video call. I will just call in if that is the case. I probably should not have told them about our plans while the stay-at-home order is in effect. However, my interpretation is that we may go to see family provided we take all the correct precautions and we are performing work that cannot be done from home.

Chapter 16 – MAY 2021

May 1

We spent the day getting ready for our trip.

A PSW called me to discuss my mom’s condition. I told her that I will not be able to visit her for the next two weeks but I will call for daily updates.

May 3

I recorded the news.

Ontario is reporting an increase in the number of Covid-19 cases as new infections jump back above 3,700 on Sunday, which is 360 more cases than what was reported on Saturday.

Ontario's test positivity rate also increased on Sunday to eight and half percent. In the previous twenty-four-hour period, 45,301 tests were completed.

Ontario's test positivity rate had remained below eight per cent the past four days.

The number of people in intensive care units dropped slightly on Sunday, after reaching nine hundred on the previous day.

There are now 895 people receiving care in intensive care due to Covid-19. Of those, 615 are breathing with the assistance of a ventilator.

As of Sunday, there are 1961 people hospitalized due to Covid-19 in Ontario.

On Sunday, Health officials reported 1198 new Covid-19 cases in Toronto, 797 in Peel Region, 306 in York Region, and 232 in Durham Region.

The other health regions reporting new caseloads in the triple digits include Hamilton, Ottawa, Simcoe-Muskoka, Niagara, and Halton Region.

Forty percent of Ontario population have received one dose of Covid-19 vaccine. Seniors, vulnerable persons and medical workers make up the majority of the vaccinated.

By the end of May, everyone over the age of eighteen will qualify for the vaccine.

Health officials warn that although over 175,000 individuals in Simcoe Muskoka have received their first dose of a Covid-19 vaccine, until everyone is fully protected, we must continue to:

stay home if sick,

keep a distance,

wear a mask,

wash your hands,

do not gather outside your immediate household, and avoid contact.

These precautions are necessary due to the uncertainty regarding the vaccines ability to protect against the Covid-19 variants, lack of evidence that vaccinated individuals do not spread Covid-19 and the length of time of vaccine effectiveness.

During the uncertainty of the pandemic, it is important to take care of your emotional health. The W.H.O. provides the following tips:

Try not to judge how you're feeling. All feelings are valid and they can change each day. Remember that people deal with change in different ways.

Give yourself breaks from checking the news. Seek out positive news when you can.

Reach out to friends and family to hear a familiar voice and feel close when you're not together.

Exercising, eating healthy foods and getting a good night of sleep can support overall health.

Do activities you enjoy easing stress and anxiety.

Set goals for yourself with a daily or weekly routine."

The co-Chair of the JET called me about our trip up north. She said that she was disappointed that I was ignoring the stay-at-home order. I told her that we will be staying in our RV and taking every precaution. Regardless, our son needs us, and we will not let him down. She was clearly not happy with me.

After dinner, my husband's youngest sister called. Her husband's sister and his best friend both died of aggressive cancer during the week. Due to the pandemic policies, he could not visit either of them in the hospital and there will not be any funerals. He was understandably extremely upset, depressed and has resorted to abusing alcohol.

May 4

I went to visit mom before we left for our trip. She was awake in her chair and had some juice, tea and cookies. I did not tell her that I was going up north for a couple of weeks. She had no idea that our son and his wife lost their jobs and were forced to move to Barry's Bay during the pandemic. We planned to take our RV to their new home and help them set up a new automotive repair shop. I just gave her a kiss and hug before I left and said I will be back. When I turned to look at her as I opened the door, she was hugging her doll and smiling at me. It broke my heart.

May 5

I read in the news that local public health units used things like prizes, food vouchers, laptop draws, walk-in access and "skip-the-line" clinic promotions to encourage youth vaccination in the summer. There are mobile vaccination vehicles offering the homeless incentives to get the shot.

Proof of vaccination was rewarded by entry into restaurants, spas, cinemas, planes, trains and boats.

Unvaccinated individuals are refused access to any of the public venues.

This coercion falls into a gray area. It is not illegal to coerce someone to get an approved drug. It is illegal to coerce clinical trial participants into receiving an experimental product. Since the mRNA vaccines were released under the Emergency Act before they had adequate safety and effectiveness data, mandates and coercion should be considered illegal or at least unethical.

May 7

My younger brother called after dinner to discuss Mother's Day. He and my younger sister are not planning to visit mom because they are not prepared to get tested for Covid-19. In addition, they would need to drive from Toronto and only be allowed to visit for one hour. I told him that she probably would either be asleep or if awake, would not recognize them. I informed him that Tom and I are not in Orillia and will not see her for Mother's Day. I plan to make it up to her when we return home next week. I did not tell him where we were and he did not ask.

May 9

It is Mother's Day.

I tried to call mom, but she did not answer.

Our son came to the shop and picked us up from our RV at 4:00 pm. We drove to Combermere to get pizza pies. No one was wearing a mask, and no one was asked for proof of vaccination.

In January 2021, Barry's Bay Renfrew area was considered a hot spot with 27 cases and an outbreak in a local nursing home. There have been no recent reports of Covid-19 cases since then.

We took the pies to his house. What a spectacular view. We ate dinner on their deck overlooking the lake. After dinner we explored their grounds and watched our son create a fire pit from rocks on the property, while our grandson did some fishing off the dock with his dog by his side. We were back at the RV by 8:00 pm. I could not ask for a nicer Mother's Day – one I cannot talk about because of the stay-at-home order.

I attempted to contact mom one more time with no success. I doubt anyone else spoke to her and I am so worried about her.

May 10

I recorded the news and used the information I found on the Simcoe Muskoka Ministry of Health website.

"Help stop the spread.

Covid-19 can be a deadly disease. You can take actions to help stop the spread:

Only travel if it's essential and isolate for fourteen days if you do.

Stay home – save lives and don't put others at risk.

Practise physical distancing – stay two metres away from anyone who is not in your household.

Wash your hands with soap and water thoroughly and often.

Learn about face coverings – how to use, clean and dispose.

Get the facts about Covid-19 – basics, symptoms and treatment.

Get sector-specific resources to prevent Covid-19 in the workplace.

Find out about the declaration of emergency and provincewide stay-at-home order.

Find your public health unit and check their website for details about vaccination in designated hot spots.

As Covid-19 cases continue to rise at an alarming rate, a declaration of emergency and province wide Stay-at-Home order are in effect as of Thursday, April 8, at 12:01 a.m.

The Covid-19 Response Framework (colour-coded zones) is paused.

We must all follow temporary restrictions and public health and workplace safety measures.

The Stay-at-Home order is in place until May 19, 2021, as the province continues to deal with the impacts of Covid-19.

This means you must stay at home. You should only go out for necessities, such as:

the grocery stores or pharmacy,

health care services (including going to medical appointments or getting vaccinated), outdoor exercise or walking pets in your community, work that cannot be done remotely, and childcare or school.

You are not allowed to gather indoors or outdoors with anyone you do not live with, except one other person from outside of the household that lives alone.

Limit close contact to only members of your household (the people you live with). If you live alone, you can have close contact with only one other household.

You must stay at least two metres apart from everyone else and wear a mask or face covering during permitted events such as a wedding, funeral or religious service, rite or ceremony.

If you do not follow these rules for gatherings:

Organizers may be fined a minimum of $10,000.

Each attendee may receive a $750 ticket.

Enforcement personnel may break up the gathering or temporarily close the premises.

If a police officer or other provincial offences officer has reason to suspect that you are participating in an organized public event or social gathering, they may require you to provide information to ensure you are complying with restrictions.

This additional enforcement tool will only be in effect during the Stay-at-Home order.

Drive-in services are permitted.

Do not travel outside your region or the province unless necessary.

You may be asked to identify yourself to a provincial offences officer if they believe you have not complied with certain orders under the Health Protection and Promotion Act, Emergency Management and Civil Protection Act, Reopening Ontario (A Flexible Response to Covid-19) Act

If the officer finds you are not following the orders, you may be fined. The set fines are:

$750 for individuals who are not following an order,

$1,000 for corporations that are not following an order, and

$1,000 for anyone who prevents an enforcement officer from exercising their powers or performing their duties to enforce the orders.

Maximum fines are:

$100,000 for an individual,

$500,000 for a director or officer of a corporation, and

$10 million for a corporation.

Failure to follow the rules could also result in prosecution or even a year in jail.

As of April 19, 2021, all publicly funded and private elementary and secondary schools are teaching classes remotely.

In-person learning is available for students with special education needs who cannot be accommodated through remote learning. Contact your school board for more information.

Licensed childcare centres and home-based childcare services for non-school-aged children are open with enhanced health and safety measures.

Before and after school programs are closed.

Emergency childcare for school-aged children is available free of charge for eligible health care, public safety and other frontline workers.

Most non-essential retailers may open for curbside pickup and delivery only, by appointment between 7:00 a.m. to 8:00 p.m. for sales, with delivery allowed between 6:00 a.m. and 9:00 p.m.

Grocery stores, convenience stores and pharmacies can open for in-person shopping at a maximum capacity of 25%.

All other establishments must remain closed."

As I read the news into the recording device, I felt a wave of guilt. I was telling people to stay home and not travel and we had just done the complete opposite. I am certain that many others would use their own judgement and ignore the order. Hopefully, we will not get caught.

In preparation for the meeting today, the secretary of the JET sent me an email with instructions for Zoom meetings by phone. The meeting focused on a patient survey I suggested about virtual care, mental health resources, home care, communication, twenty-four hours seven days a week access, hospital post-release monitoring, primary care, dental care, vision care and hearing care.

May 11

I chaired the PFAC meeting using the phone only. We discussed the patient survey and made several recommendations to the JET.

My mom's physiotherapist called to discuss her condition. He visited her today and noticed several bed sores. He will order a new air mattress and seat cushion for her wheelchair to prevent more bed sores. Hopefully, these improvements will also help with her chronic pain.

May 13

Our son asked us to stay for another week so I can look after our grandson. The schools are closed and he and his wife are busy setting up their new business. There is no daycare open in their area and his in-laws just returned from travelling in Europe and are under quarantine. The weather has been warm so we will remain outdoors at our son's new shop during the day and our grandson will go home with his mom and dad at night.

May 14

The CCRA Home Care Nurse called me to discuss mom. She is not doing very well since I stopped visiting and keeps asking for me. They will try to send a nurse a few times during the week to check on her. I expressed my sincere gratitude knowing that they were going out of their way to help her.

May 15

Today, Astra Zeneca reported that their Covid-19 viral vector vaccine is linked to blood clots. They are delaying distribution until they have more information. That is a shame because it is not a mRNA vaccine and was manufactured using a more traditional vaccine method.

Today, there are currently 2,300 Covid-19 cases in Ontario with eight of them in Orillia. There are no cases here in Barrys Bay even though people are not staying home, not wearing masks and tourists keep arriving from Toronto. We are now relieved that we decided to come here.

May 16

It is Sunday and the shop is closed so I walked the two kilometers to the Metro store in town and picked up one week's worth of groceries. I had just returned to the RV when the nurse from mom's home called. Mom is much worse. She has not taken anything by mouth for five days. They are requesting permission to discontinue all her medications because they are worried that she may choke on the pills. I agreed, although I knew that meant that she would not get any pain relief. She said that the home has given me permission to visit anytime without the need for a Covid-19 test. This does not sound good at all.

I spoke to Mom's doctor thirty minutes later to confirm my wishes to remove all medications. He will order a symptom relief kit and send it to the home. The kit will include injectable morphine.

I called our son to let him know that we need to return home tomorrow. I asked him and our grandson to come today so we can say good-bye. We do not know when we will be able to come back.

I decided not to call my brother or sister to let them know yet. They cannot visit or do anything to help, so there is no need to upset them any sooner than necessary. Mom may rally again as she did before.

I recorded the news for tomorrow.

"Some good news.

The number of new cases of Covid-19 in Ontario is dropping.

As the Stay-at-Home order appears to be working it will remain in effect until at least June 2 and all current restrictions will continue to apply.

At the end of the Stay-at-home order, there will remain some restrictions. For example, the Board of Education is considering whether children will return to their classrooms after the Stay-at-home order ends in June.

More good news.

Over 50% of all Ontario residents have received one dose of Covid-19 vaccine. Everyone who received a vaccine requiring two doses will receive their second dose sixteen weeks after their first dose.

Those who received their first dose of Astra Zeneca vaccine may need to wait more than sixteen weeks to receive their second dose. In fact, they may receive a different type of vaccine for their second dose. Health officials are considering their options and will contact affected individuals with their decision.

If you have received a Covid-19 vaccine, and specifically the Astra Zeneca vaccine, and are experiencing any new health issues, you should contact your doctor to report them. As with any vaccine, although serious side effects are rare, they may be life threatening if not treated immediately.

There have been reports that individuals who have received one dose of any Covid-19 vaccine have tested positive for Covid-19 or its variants. Fortunately, the majority experienced mild symptoms. Even if you have been vaccinated, if you become infected with Covid-19 you can spread it to others who have not yet received any vaccine or are not adequately protected by the vaccine they received. For these reasons, it is very important that even if you have received one or two doses of vaccine, you continue to wear a mask when in public and to keep your distance from everyone. These measures are in effect until most Ontarians have been vaccinated and the number of new cases has been drastically decreased."

May 17

We are getting ready to leave for home this morning. I conferenced mom's doctor with the nurse. Things are progressing quickly with calls from the CCAC, the local hospice and mom's assisted living facility. Mom will be transferred tomorrow to Mariposa House Hospice in Orillia. They will be able to take better care of her there.

During the drive home, I called my brother to provide an update. He was understandably upset and promised to inform our sister. I spoke to our son and informed him that his grandma will be going to the Hospice. He was upset that he could not come down to provide support. The good news is that he is already booked with jobs the entire week and his in-laws agreed to look after our grandson until the weekend.

May 18

At 8:00 am I went to see mom and ordered an ambulance to transport her to the hospice. I packed several personal items to take with us, including the doll, a teddy bear, my dad's urn and his photo to keep her company. We arrived at the hospice at 2:15 pm. It is a lovely place with kind and efficient staff. The Director, who is also a friend of mine, met us at the front door. I stayed with mom until 5:30 pm as the nurses accessed her condition and gave her some morphine. They will not give her anything to eat or drink until they are certain she can swallow. They will not provide life support, only pain management. Those are the instructions mom prepared last year when she was of sound mind.

May 19

I visited mom from 8:30 am until 11:45 am. She seemed about the same as yesterday. However, she did appear to know that I was there. I went home for lunch with Tom. While I was home, I cancelled mom's phone, cable, foot care, incontinence care and her medications. I returned to the hospice at 1:30 pm and came home at 5:00 pm. She appeared free of pain. Otherwise, there was no change in her condition, and she had not eaten or drank anything since arriving. I felt guilty that I could not give her anything to drink. The nurse warned me about the risk of choking or inhaling liquid if I attempted to give her a drink. She complained that she was thirsty and all I could do was moisten her lips with coconut oil they provided.

May 20

Mom was communicating this morning when I arrived at 8:30 am. She said that she was in pain. The nurse immediately installed a morphine port in her tummy. Within minutes she was comfortably asleep. I brought my lunch and a thermos of tea so I could stay all day with her.

I chatted with the Director of the hospice. She said that mom could stay there for three months and if she needs to exceed the three months, they could extend it. The provincial government covers the cost of care if it is warranted. The hospice facility relies on donations. She said that the hospice is not just for the dying, it is also for those who cannot adequately manage their pain and do not want life-support. If she survived the three months she could be placed directly into a long-term care home. She need never go to a hospital. That is all good information to know.

May 21

I left for mom's at 8:00 am. She appears comfortable so I sent some photos to my brother and sister. Our son called to just talk so I was not alone.

I went home for lunch at noon and returned at 1:00 pm. Mom remained comfortable all afternoon and I left her sleeping at 4:00 pm.

It is over thirty degrees centigrade, so I took a drive around the port on my way home. The boat launches and marinas will open this weekend and that will make a lot of people very happy.

May 22

This is the beginning of the Victoria long weekend.

I visited mom again this morning. I don't know how much longer she can survive with no fluids or sustenance. She was comfortable all morning, so I went home for lunch. When I returned, they had given her more morphine. Her skin feels cool and her breathing is shallow. I think that we are getting near the end.

I left at 4:00 pm. The retirement home called me at dinnertime and said that they needed mom's room emptied by the beginning of next month. They need to paint before the next resident can move in. We went after dinner to start organizing her things. I spoke to mom's PSW about the hospital bed, the motorized recliner and her clothes. I wondered if any of the residents could use them. She would distribute the clothes and ask around about the bed and chair. When no one was looking she gave me a hug. Before she turned away, I saw the tracks of tears running into her mask.

May 23

I had a very restless night and decided to go earlier today to see mom. When I arrived at 7:30 am, the nurse told me that mom had received two doses of morphine during the night and was showing signs of organ failure this morning. When I entered mom's room, I called out to her: "I'm here mom" as was my practice for the past ten years. I heard her take a breath and then there was silence. I went to her and put my face next to her mouth and nose. I could not feel anything. She was cool to the touch and her skin was blotchy. She was gone.

I removed my mask and kissed her on her forehead. Then I waited a few minutes to compose myself before going to fetch the nurse. I told her that mom had just passed. She was shocked and said that she was breathing normally when I arrived at the front door. I said, "She waited for me to arrive." That brought tears to the nurse's eyes.

My dad did the same thing when he was dying of cancer in a hospital ten years ago. My mother, brother and sister were already there when I arrived, and he was still breathing when I came through the door. He took his last breath just minutes after I took my place beside his bed. My mom said, "He waited for you to arrive".

I was comforted that mom had me by her side in the end and was not forced to suffer and die alone in a hospital like so many unfortunate souls over the past year. Transferring her to a hospice was the best decision I ever made. It allowed her to die in comfort and dignity. I wish I had known about these wonderful places when my dad's time was near.

I called my husband, my son and my brother to give them the news. My brother will call my sister. She is a very emotional person, and I cannot deal with her right now. I asked my brother to also call the rest of our family. Then I sat beside mom holding her hand to wait for the staff to take care of her.

I watched as the PSW opened the door to the balcony and then gently wash her. I asked why she did that. The PSW said that in some cultures they believe opening a door or window allows the soul or spirit to leave the room freely. The washing is a last act of care.

When she completed her ritual, she put a clean nightgown on mom and covered her with a homemade quilt someone had donated. Her head remained uncovered.

Mom's doctor came at 11:00 am to sign the death certificate. The funeral home came at 11:30 and placed her on a gurney and covered her with the quilt. Everyone was so compassionate and spent time to express their condolences and to ask if I was ok. They confirmed that transferring my mom to the hospice was the right decision.

The staff conducted a Walk of Life to the front door while playing the piece I requested, Bette Medler's the Wind Beneath My Wings.

In the lobby, we passed a beautiful painting of butterflies rising to the heavens. The Director explained that butterflies represent the soul, transformation and resurrection, marking the transition from physical form to a spiritual existence. Often viewed as messengers from the afterlife, butterflies represent the soul's liberation and rebirth, comforting the bereaved by symbolizing continued existence. I had never heard this before, and it gave me comfort now.

After mom was placed into the hearse, I went back to the room to collect my dad's urn and photo and told him that mom will be back with us soon. I followed the hearse to the funeral home and finalized the arrangements for my mom's cremation. I returned home at 1:00 pm feeling numb. There will be no viewing and no funeral.

I had to witness and endure mom's final journey alone. The pandemic took the support from her, me, her family and friends. I will never find it in myself to forgive the government and the medical community for their lack of empathy and inability to find solutions to everyday struggles.

Mom's PSW at the assisted living facility called to express her condolences and I told her that we will meet her tomorrow in mom's former room to look at the bed and chair. In the meantime, she will go through the clothes and take anything that others may use.

May 24

I extracted information from the local health unit and without much thought recorded the news.

"Happy Victoria Day from the City of Orillia!

A reminder that all City of Orillia facilities are closed and services provided by phone or email are not available today. Orillia Transit is not running and there is no curbside collection today. Collection will be delayed by one day for the remainder of the week.

The second-dose emails have been sent to those who received their first dose of the Covid-19 vaccine at a community clinic prior to March 17 AND did not have a second dose appointment scheduled (or had one cancelled). If you have not received the email, the instructions and booking link are now on the Simco Muskoka health unit website.

NOTE: You must book your appointment for the week your second dose is due. If you book earlier, you will be turned away at the clinic and risk having your second dose delayed further.

The province announced that as of May 22 outdoor limits for social gatherings and organized public events is expanded to five people. Remember, all other public health and workplace safety measures under the provincewide emergency brake are still in effect, and protective public health measures still need to be practiced.

We know you are tired, but with forty-four percent of our population having received their first dose of the Covid-19 vaccine, there is a light at the end of the tunnel.

So, for now, even if you have been vaccinated, please continue to follow public health measures.

Being vaccinated doesn't mean that you can't get Covid-19. You can. However, the antibodies you have from the vaccine should keep you from getting very sick with the illness.

In fact, some individuals that had both doses and were going for a procedure at the hospital, tested positive for the virus despite being asymptomatic. Although the vaccine should keep you from becoming infectious, you can still theoretically spread the virus even once you are vaccinated.

Protect yourself even if you have had the vaccine and continue to wear your mask, distance and follow public health guidelines.

We have lots of vaccine coming now and anyone over the age of eighteen is allowed to get vaccinated. It is hoped by the end of the summer anyone over the age of twelve can get vaccinated.

The government is hopeful that this will be the final lockdown because of vaccines.

Public Health Ontario has reported 1,691 new cases of Covid-19 yesterday.

Due to the Victoria Day holiday, there will be no provincial Covid-19 numbers posted today. Reporting will resume tomorrow."

We started taking mom's things home. The PSW came with her son to take the motorized chair to an elderly neighbour with mobility issues. We were happy to see it go to good use.

May 25

I chaired a PFAC meeting this morning and attended a JET meeting. Everyone knew that I had returned home to be with my mom and of her passing. The Director of the Mariposa House is a member of the COHT, and she informed them of my situation. The first few minutes of the meeting were spent communicating their condolences. I was very touched.

I went to the funeral home to pick up some paperwork and to approve her urn before going back to mom's room to do more organizing.

I am feeling lost without mom to visit every day. I have been her essential caregiver for the past ten years and now that she and dad are both gone, and our son is married with his own life, I feel like an orphan with no purpose.

May 26

We went to mom's and continued sorting out her things. We took four bags of things that are in no condition to be donated to the dump. I called the store where we bought the hospital bed last year to see if they would buy it back. They will not.

May 27

The room is still full of mom's furniture. I called several movers in the area. No one is available until June 9. I spoke to the retirement home, and they said I could keep the room until then.

May 29

We brought the hospital bed home in pieces. I listed it, the transfer chair and walker on Kijiji. I received a notice from the website that medical devices cannot be listed and sold using that platform.

Everything is now packed and ready to be donated. All the furniture is ready for the movers. We took the clothes to Value Village and were told that they cannot accept donations until the middle of June, when the lockdown is over. We had to take everything home with us.

May 31

I prepared and recorded the news.

"There have been 147 new cases reported to the Simcoe Muskoka District Health Unit for the past week. There were 303 new cases reported to the health unit in the week of May 16th, thirteen percent lower than the 348 cases reported for the week of May 9th.

There were 25 Covid-19 deaths in April, double the 12 Simcoe Muskoka residents who died from Covid-19 in March. There have been eighteen Covid-19 deaths so far in May among Simcoe

Muskoka residents.

With most Ontario residents experiencing "pandemic fatigue," the Ontario Medical Association has offered several opinions and insights on how people might cope with changes in our lives when the pandemic comes to an end.

For some it could be party time. For others it will be a time of difficulty and mistrust.

"It has been fourteen months since the World Health Organization declared a pandemic; fourteen very long months for everyone. And now people all over the globe are asking themselves how will it end? Because we know pandemics always end.

Will we go back to the lives we lived before, or have things changed to the point that some of our behaviours have changed forever.

A panel of medical experts gathered on Wednesday to comment on what Ontario residents can expect in terms of physical health and mental health among themselves and family members. They predicted "that COVD is going to be around for the foreseeable future and probably for the long-term."

Here are some of the highlights:

Despite the vaccines, it will not be enough to eliminate every case. Covid-19 will hopefully become treatable as an "outpatient" disease.

What is required, is for the virus to be stopped for a long period, long enough that there is no infection of other mammals such as dogs or mice or some other species.

The virus might continue to evolve into something like a seasonal influenza that changes over time. If that becomes the case, Covid-19 would no longer be regarded as seriously as it is now, but neither would it be "a trivial disease."

It will be up to the infectious disease professionals to determine exactly when the pandemic is over, and that will inspire a small portion of the population to immediately act like nothing ever happened.

Another part of society, roughly thirty to fifty percent, would gradually and cautiously slide back into a sense of normalcy and will be accepting of some changes.

Maybe ten to twenty percent will have difficulty moving forward. They would remain overly fearful and would avoid others.

There has been an increase in serious mental health issues that affect people's moods, cause sleep disturbances, lack of interest, lack of energy, concentration problems, feelings of guilt and worthlessness and levels of anxiety to the point where people cannot function. Those suffering from medical health issues will require both medical and community support.

In the meantime, we need to all do our part in keeping Covid-19 at bay."

My husband and I will be in the group of hermits. Not because we are fearful. It is more that we are disappointed in humanity. The government consists of sheep in wolves' clothing, and the rest are the sheep just following orders. Academia is mainly to blame. On the whole, it now teaches students what to think rather than how to think. A small percentage challenge everything and those are labelled conspiracy theorists.

Chapter 17

JUNE 2021

June 1

I sent an email to BANAC to remind them of our meeting on July 13 to discuss the PFAC. They requested that I send a copy of my presentation and my questions before the meeting.

The movers called and cancelled the June 9 appointment. Now we have no one to help us move mom's furniture from her room. We decided to post an announcement on the local market site on Facebook that the furniture will be in the parking lot tomorrow at 4:00 pm and it is available free on a first-come basis.

June 2

We went to mom's room and brought all her furniture down from the second floor. None of the staff could help us due to the lock down rules. We struggled but managed to get it all out of the building and into the parking lot. At 4:00 pm, three people showed up and took most of the items. We loaded the remaining pieces into our trailer for transport home.

The manager came to check on our progress. She told me that I needed to take the relief kit with me. I said that the CCAC had ordered it and because it contained controlled substances they needed to come and retrieve it. I asked her for the tax form, and she said I would get it when the room is completely cleaned out. Can you imagine being held hostage like that?

The funeral home called to let me know that mom's remains were ready to be picked up. At least that part of the process is efficient. Things seem to move much faster when a person is dead than when they are alive.

June 3

I went this morning to bring mom home to be together with dad. They are both now resting on my bookshelf and I feel them watching over me. Their wish was that I co-sprinkle their ashes near their cottage in Muskoka. I will fulfill their final wish after the pandemic is over. In the meantime, their presence will bring me comfort.

A couple came to pick up the last few pieces of mom's furniture. While we were chatting in our driveway, I heard a crash and a scream. I ran across the street to our neighbour's backyard. The ninety-year-old man was lying unconscious on the ground with a ladder beside him. His wife saw me from the window and came running out of the back door. Tom and the couple joined us seconds later. The elderly man had apparently fallen off the ladder and landed against a wooden fence post.

I offered to call 911 or take him to the hospital. By that time, he had regained consciousness. He declined to go due to fear of the hospital. I told his wife to keep him awake for the rest of the day and to let me know if there is any change in his behaviour.

I returned home with my husband and the couple. None of them could figure out how I knew to run over to our neighbour's backyard because they had not heard anything. I said that I am always listening and looking out for our elderly neighbours. The man has dementia and is always doing unsafe things. When I heard the crash and scream, I just knew that he was in trouble.

June 4

I spoke to the neighbour, and she said that her husband appeared fine this morning. He had a large cut on his head and elbow, so she applied bandages to both. He has dementia, so it is difficult to know if he is not behaving normal. The fact that he was on a ladder attempting to get up on the roof at the age of ninety, demonstrates a lack of judgement and abnormal behaviour. He really needs to be in a long-term-care home, but I would not wish that on anyone.

June 5

We finished cleaning out mom's room and brought the remaining items home to store in our garage.

June 6

A young man came from Kingston to pick up the hospital bed for his mom. They had just arrived from India and did not have very much. His mom had suffered a stroke and has difficulty getting out of bed. He was very pleased with it and grateful. It felt good to give it to someone in need.

We are planning to hold a garage sale when it is allowed to unload the remaining items.

June 7

I recorded the news.

"Effective June 2 the provincial declaration of emergency and stay-at-home order expired. All other existing measures and restrictions will remain in place until the province is ready to enter Step One of Ontario's Roadmap to Reopen. The province expects to enter Step One the week of June 14, but this date has not yet been confirmed.

There have been 113 new cases reported in the Simcoe Muskoka district for the past week. There were 207 cases reported on the week of May 23rd, thirty-two percent lower than the 305 cases reported for the week of May 16th.

There was eighteen

Covid-19 deaths in May among Simcoe Muskoka residents, which was lower than the 25 deaths in April.

Hugs are back! Ontario loosening restrictions at long-term care homes.

Starting June 9, you can briefly hug a long-term care resident, whether you are vaccinated or not.

And, if both the resident and visitor are fully vaccinated, hand holding and close physical contact will be permitted as well.

The new directive also allows long-term care residents who are fully immunized to leave the home for day and overnight trips starting June 9.

Residents with mobility limitations or health conditions that make participating in outdoor visits highly unlikely or impossible may also now have one general visitor at a time inside the long-term care home, in addition to an essential caregiver.

Ontario cites high levels of vaccination in long-term care homes as the reason for the change.

Forty years ago, the first cases of AIDS were reported in the US

On June 5, 1981, a curious report about five young gay men across Los Angeles had been diagnosed with an unusual lung infection and two of them had died.

It was the first time that Acquired Immune Deficiency Syndrome (AIDS) -- the devastating advanced-stage of Human Immunodeficiency Virus (HIV) infection that would go on to claim the lives of more than thirty-two million people globally -- was reported in the US.

Days after the initial report hit the newspapers, the Centers for Disease Control (CDC) learned of more such cases in gay men. Not only did those men have lung infections, but they also had other secondary infections, among them a rare and aggressive cancer known as Kaposi's sarcoma.

About a month after that first report, twenty-six gay men across New York and California had similar diagnoses -- a number that would increase exponentially.

Saturday marked the fortieth anniversary of the nation's first reported cases of AIDS. More than 700,000 people in the US have died of the disease since then -- and though medical advancements have drastically changed the prognosis for HIV/AIDS patients.

In the early eighties HIV/AIDS was considered a death sentence.

The tide started to turn in the late eighties and nineties, as more effective therapies became available and transformed what it meant for an individual to live with HIV.

Despite the US setting a goal in 1997 to find an HIV vaccine within ten years, four decades later, there is still no vaccine.

I finalized the agenda for the PFAC meeting tomorrow and sent it out to the members.

I attended a JET meeting and based on the experience with my mom,

I proposed that a Working Group be established to improve access to PSWs and homecare. We need an alternative to LTC homes. The government could invest in home care rather than construction. Smaller congregate living spaces with personalized care would be preferable to the current LTC homes. The JET will bring my suggestion to the COHT for further consideration. I doubt that it will get much traction because there is big money in the retirement and LTC business. I have a habit of following the money, and in this case, it leads to the bank accounts of investors.

June 8

I chaired the PFAC meeting and the following topics were discussed.

During the JET meeting on Monday June 7th, I raised the concern that getting quality care in LTC facilities or at home, is a challenge. There is substandard care in some of these facilities and an increasing number of people do not want to go into LTC or to assisted living homes. We need to rethink how to care for frail seniors at home.

An understanding of how to navigate between different organizations created by each political party is required. They all co-exist and this creates confusion for the public, inefficiencies and unnecessary cost. We need clarity on each organization and what they do.

The mandate of Ontario Health Teams is to bring together all the different pieces to make our healthcare system easier to navigate for patients and families. So far, this is not working.

I suggested that we need an article in one of the three news venues in Orillia. A reporter could conduct research on the overlap of the OHT and other government organizations. They could also research the handling of the pandemic. The PFAC could provide support for the article which could cover patient interactions with the health care system, virtual access to medical records, clinical planning, communication and why the PFAC is important. We could use the article to recruit new members.

It was decided that I would speak to reporters about the article.

We will also request from the Ontario Ministry of Health, clarification of the roles and responsibilities of the Community Care Access Centers (CCAC), the Local Health Integration Network (LHIN), Home and Community Care (HCC) and Ontario Health Teams (OHT). They all co-exist with similar mandates.

June 9

I finalized the PFAC recruitment documents and the minutes of yesterday's meeting. I sent emails to several reporters about the potential article. One of the reporters replied immediately and arranged to call me on Friday to discuss the article.

The government must have read my mind. I received a proposed new regulation from Ontario Health to review and provide comments. It puts the responsibility for Home Care in the hands of the LHIN and then to the OHT when it is fully formed. All LTC homes and Home Care companies would tender and if approved, contract with the LHIN who would pay for their services. The LHIN would also be responsible for monitoring the quality of services. This is a great initiative and one that the PFAC would support.

June 10

I read and summarized the Ontario Health document. I spoke to a few of the JET members about it and recommended that the COHT create a budget for and fill a PFAC Quality position to conduct audits of programs via patient interviews. I sent them the following position paper.

Background: To measure the impact of system changes, specifically those implemented in response to PFAC recommendations or community surveys, a Quality Plan should be put into place. This plan should outline the methods used to measure changes both quantitatively and qualitatively using Quality Indicators. The Quality Plan should be developed and implemented by impartial Quality staff.

Written procedures for conducting PFAC business should be prepared to ensure consistency and transparency. A few examples of activities are Terms of Reference, Minutes of meetings, Quality Plan, community information collection, patient engagement, confidentiality agreement, volunteer contract, reimbursement procedure and compensation policy.

Documents created for and by the PFAC should be version controlled and retained. This is especially important when changes occur in staff and Council members. We need to ensure that everyone is using the most recent approved documents.

Recommendation: The Quality component of the PFAC activities requires a dedicated Quality lead with Quality background and training. It is an ongoing function that should be implemented as soon as possible.

I sent emails to two more reporters and heard back from everyone. It appears that the topic generated much interest. I will chat with each of them tomorrow.

June 11

I sent an email to the JET members with a summary that I prepared of the new Home Care regulations.

I spoke with three reporters, and they all agreed to do an article on the Ontario Health System.

June 14

I recorded the news. There was not much in the way of health news, so I created some suggestions for seniors to stay healthy.

"June is Seniors Month

Seniors can stay active and healthy in the heat of the summer if they exercise safely.

Older adults may face additional factors that could increase risk during extreme heat, such as chronic conditions, social isolation, or medications that interfere with the body's cooling mechanisms.

Planning and modifying your physical activity can reduce your risk. Consider going for a walk early in the morning or during the evening.

Staying connected by exercising with others has many benefits such as motivating you to get moving.

Drinking more water is important. By the time you feel thirsty you are already dehydrated. So, drink plenty of water before and during exercise.

Try not to expect the usual performance from your body during extreme heat and allow your body to recover and cool down after heat exposure.

Watch for signs of heat illness. These include dizziness or fainting, nausea or vomiting, headache or rapid breathing and heartbeat. If you have any of these signs move to a cool place and drink plenty of water right away.

Retirees can benefit from engaging in their community.

Share your passion. Your unique skills and interests can bring joy and support to others. Communicating your passion can help keep your community engaged, fight feelings of loneliness and create lasting friendships.

Create a connection. Reach out to a friend by picking up the phone to check on how they are feeling.

Get involved. Ask local organizations how you can contribute. If you are in a retirement home, a resident's council is a great way to get together to plan activities, share ideas, talents, wisdom and develop helpful suggestions for the home.

Spread positivity. If you have had an opportunity to give back, share the news with friends, family and your retirement community. You may inspire others to make a difference.

Positive Things the Pandemic Has Changed for Good

Working from home has become a positive alternative for many types of work.

Staying in touch by video calls with family and friends allows more frequent gatherings, especially with those who live far away.

Virtual care without long wait times in the office has improved access to health care.

Travel by plane has been significantly reduced which has decreased air pollution. Hopefully this will continue.

More people are growing and shopping for food locally. Farmer markets have become very popular for food and crafts.

June 15

One of the local newspapers published an article about the PFAC. They used most of the information I had prepared for them. I sent a copy of the article to the JET and PFAC members.

June 16

The Chair of the JET called to touch base regarding messaging. We had a good discussion. It was agreed that I will tell the COHT members at the next meeting that I am working with local reporters to create a series of articles about the Ontario Health System and the COHT in support of PFAC recruitment. I will ask if any of the COHT member organizations have an objection to being included or mentioned in the articles. The theme of the series is who comprises the COHT, accomplishments in the face of the pandemic, future goals, and the importance of patient and caregiver input.

I will schedule several PFAC meetings to finalize the member recruitment strategy, which will include, community outreach, application forms, interview process, meetings, minutes and action logs.

In the afternoon, I received several calls from the public asking for more information about the PFAC after reading the article.

June 17

A few more people called to obtain more information about the PFAC. Apparently, the article is helping with the community outreach.

I attended the COHT meeting and we discussed the PFAC. It was decided that I should postpone the meeting on July 13 with the Barrie Area Native Advisory Circle (BANAC), Health Circle until we finalize the recruitment strategy. I sent an email to BANAC apologizing for the cancellation and explaining the reasons for the delay.

June 18

The first two applications were received by me for the PFAC.

I received a response from BANAC. They agreed that August may be preferable for them because many of their members are on vacation during July.

June 19

I sent the slides approved by the JET for the Health Circle meeting to the BANAC for review prior to the meeting with them. This will provide more time for them to digest the information and should result in a productive meeting in August.

June 21

I recorded the news.

"Today is National Indigenous Peoples Day.

Volunteers sought to help improve care for seniors, an article in the Orillia Matters online newsletter.

"A group of volunteers is setting out to find ways to improve the care provided to frail seniors.

The Patient and Family Advisory Council, part of the Couchiching Ontario Health Team, is looking for more volunteers to join as it begins reaching out to frail seniors in long-term care homes, retirement homes and other settings. The volunteer work will "influence improvements in health-care navigation, virtual care, clinical management, record sharing and communications," explained PFAC volunteer and Chair Susan Langlois.

"We want to find out what areas need improving, and we will also be part of the solution," she said, noting the council will make recommendations to the COHT based on the feedback it receives from seniors.

Their interactions with the health-care system — for example, their experiences with a personal support worker (PSW) — are what the PFAC wants to learn more about.

"We can't change what the PSWs do or what the nurses do, but we can address the way they're interacting," Langlois said.

The PFAC is looking for volunteers who have had experiences with the health-care system in the past five years. They should be patients or family members who have been caregivers.

Those interested must fill out an application form and go through an interview process.

The City of Orillia and the Age-Friendly Orillia Advisory Committee have hired a consultant to conduct a Needs Assessment to determine what the people of Orillia need to improve their lives. "

I attended a JET meeting by video. We were informed that the assistant assigned to support me will be replaced by the secretary of the JET co-chair. My request for a Quality position was not included in the agenda. I mentioned the omission and was told that they have a different opinion about Quality and that they would include the topic on the agenda for the next meeting.

June 23

I organized interviews with two potential members of the PFAC.

I organized a meeting with the JET coordinator to discuss a promotion piece for the COHT.

June 24

I was asked to record the news a second time this week.

"The Ontario Premier's office just announced a change in the reopening of the province.

Starting June 30, Ontario is lifting Covid-19-related restrictions further by putting the province in the second step of its Roadmap to Reopen.

The changes to public health measures include the following allowances:

Outdoor social gatherings and organized public events with up to twenty-five people.

Indoor social gatherings and organized public events with up to five people.

Essential and other select retail permitted at fifty percent capacity.

Non-essential retail permitted at twenty-five per cent capacity.

Personal care services where face coverings can be worn at all times, and at twenty-five percent capacity and other restrictions.

Outdoor dining with up to six people per table, with exceptions for larger households and other restrictions.

Indoor religious services, rites, or ceremonies, including wedding services and funeral services permitted at up to twenty-five per cent capacity of the room.

Outdoor fitness classes limited to the number of people who can maintain three metres of physical distance.

Outdoor sports without contact or modified to avoid contact, with no specified limit on number of people or teams participating, with restrictions.

Overnight camps for children operating in a manner consistent with the safety guidelines produced by the Office of the Chief Medical Officer of Health.

Outdoor sport facilities, outdoor concert venues, theatres and cinemas, outdoor horse racing and motor speedways, and outdoor fairs, rural exhibitions, festivals are all permitted at twenty per cent capacity and with other restrictions.

According to the news release issued by the Ontario Premier's office today, Ontario will stay in Step Two for approximately twenty-one days.

On June 11, 2021, the province lifted its previous stay-at-home order/emergency brake lockdown restrictions to start Step One of the Roadmap to Reopen. At that time, the government said the province would remain in Step One for at least twenty-one days.

Volunteers are sought to help improve care for seniors.

A group of volunteers is setting out to find ways to improve the care provided to frail seniors.

The Patient and Family Advisory Council, part of the Couchiching

Ontario Health Team, is looking for more volunteers to join as it begins reaching out to frail seniors in long-term care homes, retirement homes and other settings. The volunteer work will "influence improvements in health-care navigation, virtual care, clinical management, record sharing and communications," The council will make recommendations to the COHT based on the feedback it receives from seniors.

The PFAC is looking for volunteers who have had experiences with the Simcoe health-care system in the past five years. They should be patients or family members who have been caregivers."

Most of the gathering limits seem irrational to me. The government does not have information to support their recommendations and appear to be grasping at straws. If these Roadmap to Opening recommendations came from medical advisors, I am not surprised. They need to find advisors who are virologists and infectious disease experts who created the Pandemic Influenza Plan in 2004.

The Covid-19 virus is an airborne virus, and no manner of distancing will stop its spread. If someone infectious is present, the virus can fill the room in just a few minutes. The virus will collect on all parts of the body, surfaces and cloth masks will not filter them out. Once the mask is removed, to allow eating or drinking for instance, hands will touch other parts of the body and transfer the virus to the nose and mouth.

The most important thing to do when there is a respiratory virus outbreak is to make sure that people remain home if they have symptoms and if someone is coughing or sneezing, they do so inside their bent elbow and turn away from others. Frequent hand washing was also effective in reducing spread during the SARS epidemic, which did not reach pandemic proportions.

I organized the PFAC documents and the plan for the interviews. I participated in the PFAC Network meeting at noon.

After the meeting I spoke with the JET coordinator about the need to include PFAC representatives on the COHT working groups.

PFAC needs –

more time allotted at each JET and COHT meetings to discuss our suggestions for improvements,

to visit the Shared Purpose and Values document to determine PFAC's role, and

to organize the orientation of the new PFAC members. This should include an overview of the COHT and the working groups. The Chairs of each working committee should present the overviews to ensure an accurate account.

One of the hospital volunteers called me. She had a heart attack two weeks after she received the second dose of the Pfizer vaccine. She wondered if the vaccine caused the heart attack. I said that I had seen articles referring to myocarditis after receiving a second dose of the mRNA vaccine. However, I had not seen any government or manufacturer claims that it was caused by the vaccine. I told her to speak with her physician and warned her against getting any more doses.

June 25

I prepared pre-read for the JET meeting and added items to the agenda, including the recommendation for a Quality person on the COHT, and co-design by the PFAC and COHT for all Working Groups.

I joined the Health System Performance Network (HSPN) on behalf of the COHT.

June 28

I recorded the news.

“Ontario reported 287 new Covid-19 cases on Sunday.

The update also includes 379 new recoveries and 12 deaths.

Orillia Soldiers Memorial Hospital has heightened surveillance for Covid-19 on its Integrated Medicine and Rehab Services unit. Two patients who shared a room on the forty-two-bed unit have tested positive for Covid-19.

The unit is now closed to new admissions and transfers. All other patients on the unit have tested negative, are safely quarantining in their rooms and are being monitored closely for symptoms."

June 29

I began the PFAC member interviews today. I will conduct one this afternoon and another this evening.

A publication in JAMA highlighted the risk of myocarditis after a second dose of mRNA vaccine. I assume that the government will now have to provide a warning about this risk, especially in young healthy males.

June 30

This is the first day of Step two of the Roadmap to Opening. It is such a relief to have our freedom back.

Chapter 18 – JULY 2021

July 2

I interviewed one more PFAC member this morning. I requested a copy of the COHT Confidentiality Agreement and PFAC contract from the PFAC coordinator and sent them to the potential members. I will now finalize the orientation process.

Two of the people I interviewed accepted their offers to join the PFAC. I am so relieved that I will have others to share the workload with me.

I am still waiting for confirmation from the BANAC to meet with me in August, so I sent them an email as a reminder. I have not received any comments since I sent them a copy of my presentation.

July 5

I prepared and recorded the news.

“We have now entered the second stage of Ontario’s re-opening strategy. Ontario needed to have vaccinated seventy per cent of adults with one dose of Covid-19 vaccine and twenty per cent with two doses for at least two weeks, ensuring a strong level of protection. As of June 23, over seventy-six per cent of the adult population in Ontario have received one dose of a vaccine and over twenty-nine per cent have received their second dose.

The hospital has reopened one side of their Integrated Medicine Rehab (IMRS) floor as a separate clean unit. Although not at full capacity yet, it is a good sign as their heightened surveillance continues to remain in good standing. Team members have been dedicated to either side on or two of IMRS and will remain on their dedicated side until the end of their heightened surveillance. All swabs continue to come back negative for Covid-19 and no new cases have been identified. If this continues, IMRS will return to regular operations on Sunday, July 4.

As some hospitals have taken another step toward easing visitor restrictions, the Orillia hospital is waiting until they get the all clear in regard to the heightened surveillance on IMRS before they consider any visitor modifications, which could come as early as this week. Changes under consideration would see more flexibility around the time and duration that visitors could be on site.

The Covid-19 Assessment Centre now operating out of the Rotary Place will return to the Kiwanis Building at Orillia Soldiers Memorial Hospital by Aug. 11, allowing the municipality to reopen an ice pad that the clinic is currently occupying in time for a return of recreation activities in late summer or early fall.

Established in March 2020, the Covid-19 Assessment Centre started as a drive-thru service outside the Kiwanis Building at the hospital.

As demand grew, lengthy vehicle lineups began to stretch

throughout the neighbourhoods surrounding the hospital, with wait times of up to four hours.

To improve efficiency, the centre was located at the Rotary Place with pre-booked appointments. The facility has served the community well, at times conducting more than 500 tests per day, and it provided the necessary space, accessibility and parking to provide the service safely.

The centre currently performs up to 150 tests per day, and fewer on weekends when operating hours are shorter.

Once relocated, the Assessment Center will provide both drive-thru and in-building services for as long as required.

The mass vaccination centre will continue to operate in the Orillia Room at the Rotary Place.

The Couchiching OHT is hosting a Vaccination Clinic on July 15-16 at the Rotary Place.

July 6

I chaired a PFAC meeting this morning.

There has been much completed and in progress.

The Terms of reference was completed,

the recruitment process began,

roles and responsibilities have been determined,

two new members have joined, and

two additional interested candidates have received the application form.

Many things are in process:

Orientation,

finalization of the Terms of Reference with new PFAC member input, media relations, reviewing the Patient Declaration of Values for Ontario, and seeking Indigenous partner engagement.

It was decided that the PFAC will review, amend and adopt the Ontario Health PFAC Patient Declaration of Values.

I will send the orientation package to all PFAC members.

We will discuss meeting schedule with new members at the next meeting.

I reviewed the Modernization Home and Community Care legislation and regulations from Health Ontario and sent several substantive comments to the JET. It took me four hours to do this, but I found it very interesting and encouraging. The deadline for the COHT feedback is July 15.

I finalized the PFAC minutes and sent them to the secretary for distribution to the JET.

I sent a request to the JET asking for the names and contact information of the leads to the Working Groups. I will invite them to future PFAC orientation meetings.

July 7

I began working on the PFAC orientation package which will contain the Terms of Reference, the Declaration of Values and the list of COHT members.

I sent an email to the Working Group Chairs requesting summary slides for the orientation. I also sent the PFAC Terms of Reference to each of the Chairs.

July 12

I recorded the news.

"Ontario reported 160 new Covid-19 cases on Sunday.

On Friday July 16 the province will enter the third stage of the province's re-opening strategy.

This means that we have increased the maximum number of people for outdoor gatherings from 25 to100, the number for indoor gatherings from 5 to 25 and retirement homes continue to be exempt from gathering limits.

For religious services, rites or ceremonies, including wedding and funeral services, indoor capacity of the room will increase from 25 to no limit provided physical distancing can remain two metres.

Retail capacity will increase from fifty percent for essential, including LCBO, stores, and twenty-five percent for non-essential to unlimited for both provided physical distancing of two meters is maintained. Stores in malls remain open.

Restaurants and Bars move from outdoor only dining with 6 people per table to indoor and outdoor dining with capacity limited to physical distancing of two meters and no limit on the number of people per table. Buffets will be permitted.

Personal care facilities will increase from twenty-five by appointment only and no services that require the removal of face covering to capacity limited only to permit physical distancing and may include services that require the removal of face covering.

All other facilities that were either open for outdoor only or closed during step two will be permitted to open indoors with restrictions on number of people to allow physical distancing.

The Orillia Fall Fair is very excited to announce that they are planning a one-day fair on Saturday September 11th with some of their most popular outdoor events including a demolition derby, truck & tractor pulls, inflatables, vendors, animal displays and more.

They will be in constant contact with the Simcoe Muskoka District Health Unit to maintain a safe environment for all of those in attendance and strictly adhering to all safety protocols. There will be a maximum capacity of five thousand as stated in the regulations released by the Province of Ontario. Additional information will be released as it becomes available!

The "See You on the Patio" event is now open for business every Friday and Saturday night during the summer months. This occurs on Mississauga Street in downtown Orillia.

The Orillia Farmers Market is now open at the library parking lot on Fridays from 5:00 to 9:00 pm and Saturdays from 8:00 am to 1:00 pm."

I attended a JET meeting where we discussed the series of COHT news articles. The Chair of the JET, and I agreed on the theme which I will send to the local reporters.

I received an email from BANAC. They have delayed our meeting until September. This is very disappointing and I communicated their decision to the JET.

The co-Chair of the JET sent me an email asking how many of her referrals I interviewed. I sent a response to her, the Chair and the coordinator, stating that the coordinator and I interviewed the seven individuals she referred to me and an additional seven that contacted me after reading the first article. Those fourteen resulted in three new members. Including me, we now have four. I also sent a copy of my draft PFAC Orientation package and a list of the new members to JET.

July 15

Last night, I received the JET feedback for the Modernization Home and Community Care Act with a request that I review and comment. After finishing my review, I found that many of the edits I had made earlier were missing from the final version of the document. The deadline for submission is today. At 5:30 am I sent my additional comments to the coordinator, and he called me immediately to discuss them. I concentrated my revisions on ensuring accountability, enhancing quality, and incorporating feedback from patients. He explained that the JET did not agree with the PFAC's position. I told him that it would be preferable if the PFAC could send their comments directly to Health Ontario rather than an edited version by OHT. I was once again disappointed by the lip service being paid by the COHT.

During the COHT meeting, I made a presentation to update them about the PFAC. The Chair decided to complete the article for the reporter by next week.

After the meeting, I received confirmation from the BANAC Health Circle that our meeting will be held on September 14. They have reviewed my presentation and do not have any questions or comments. I sent an email to the JET and asked if anyone else would join me during the meeting with the BANAC. Their response was that they approved the presentation and I should conduct the initial meeting myself. I hope it goes ok because if things go wrong, the responsibility for the failure will fall on me.

July 16

The Chair of the COHT sent me the draft article for review and comment. I sent my final comments to him by email.

July 19

I attended a JET meeting and followed it up with confirmation of a meeting in the middle of the week with two of the Working Group leaders.

July 20

I conducted the first PFAC orientation of new members today. It was well received and generated several questions and suggestions. The following was noted.

During the next meeting, we will review questions about OHT Overview.

We will ask the Northern PFAC Network group about their engagement with their OHT.

Members will bring suggestions for PFAC projects and priorities to the next meeting.

All members should review the Terms of Reference and Declaration of Patient Values for discussion at the next PFAC meeting.

The team agreed to attend the next COHT Collaboration Table meeting.

July 21

I had a great meeting with the first two Working Groups. They will attend the PFAC meeting on August 17 and I promised to send them background information about the three new members. I sent an email to the remaining Working Groups to encourage them to participate in PFAC meetings.

I had a pleasant phone conversation with one of the members of the JET, where we talked about PFAC strategies, the Patient Declaration, and the website.

I accepted the Chair position at the Northern PFAC Network meeting on September 29. The secretary of the COHT PFAC will take the minutes. I sent an invitation to a video conference for the participants with an agenda and pre-read.

July 26

I recorded the news.

"The Ontario government want your views on long-term care, agriculture, housing.

You are invited to let them know your ideas for resolving three of the top issues.

Long-term care: Covid-19 has surfaced significant issues affecting

Ontario's long-term care facilities – resident isolation, insufficient levels of medical staff, and inadequate personal protective equipment. There are many underlying factors - recruiting and training, wages, public vs private ownership, and registered staffing levels. Specific question for Simcoe North - What should be done to improve Long Term Care?

Agriculture: Farmers are the front line in providing food security. But too often they lack the technology, the regulations and the financial rewards to meet today's agricultural challenges. Specific question for Simcoe North - What do we need to do to make farming a successful and significant part of Simcoe North's economy?

Housing: Middle income Ontarians are finding it increasingly difficult to afford decent housing. The housing market is pricing home ownership beyond the average family's means. Too often affordable housing is simply unavailable. How should we change our approach to building and managing our housing industry to ensure we all have a safe place to live?"

A neighbour called to tell me about the communication problems she is experiencing with one of the local PSW companies. I relayed the complaint to my contact at the company.

July 27

One of the PFCA members sent an email asking if she can call me today at 3:00 pm. I confirmed that I was available. She informed me that due to mental health reasons she will need to take a leave of absence and will not be available starting today. I thanked her for the help with the committee and expressed my concern for her. I told her if she ever needs to talk to someone, I will be available but will respect her privacy.

July 29

The Chair of the JET sent me an email to inform me that the government due date for posting the Declaration of Patient Values on the COHT website was extended to November 30. Thankfully, this will provide more time to develop our website.

Chapter 19 – AUGUST 2021

August 3

I chaired a PFAC meeting and prepared the minutes.

I discussed the Engagement and Partnership Strategies with the Northern PFAC Network.

The PFAC project priorities will be discussed after the Working Groups have met with the PFAC.

The Clinical Care Redesign Working Group is scheduled to meet with the PFAC on August 17, and the Palliative Care Working Group will meet on September 14.

The Retirement Home, Long Term Care Home and Primary Care Working Groups were summarized during the public Fireside Chat on-line meeting. It was recorded and will be available for viewing on the hospital website.

The discussion of comments received regarding the Patient Declaration of Values will be postponed until the Ontario Ministry of Health provides their revised Declaration and instructions. The deadline has been extended to the end of November 2021.

The PFAC Terms of Reference were discussed. There is a concern that the PFAC is considered Advisory and this conflicts with the mandate that the system be co-designed. The potential of renaming the PFAC was entertained. Some suggestions were made – Healthcare Co-Design Council or Patient and Family Co-Design Council. It was also suggested that any COHT document include a statement that PFAC reviewed and approved it.

The PFAC should consider how it will know that it has had an impact on patient interaction and propose metrics to be included in the Indicators and Measurement document.

Invitations were received to join the next COHT meeting on August 19.

One of the next projects is to provide input into the COHT Engagement and Partnership Strategy required by the Ontario Ministry by the end of September.

The COHT and PFAC is reaching out to the Indigenous community. I was invited to make a presentation to BANAC and RAMA on Sept 14. The members of the Indigenous Health Circle include representatives from both BANAC and RAMA.

After the meeting, I reflected again on how the government boasts about the new Ontario Health Teams and how they will improve health care for all patients. Over the past twelve months, I have witnessed the introduction of many new policies and procedures that did not include patient and caregiver input. I also witnessed attacks on individuals who disagree with the direction the health care has taken. Experts have not been utilized or listened to. Only politicians, large companies and influential elites are controlling the management of the pandemic. If one follows the money, they will conclude that the actions taken only benefit the rich and powerful. Going forward, I will abandon my diplomatic approach and become a stronger advocate for patients, families and caregivers. I made a conscious decision to apply my expertise and experience to advise those who do not have the capacity to help themselves and to go public with my stand on the lockdowns, Covid-19 vaccine and mandates.

August 8

I prepared and recorded the news.

"Ontario Ramping Up Efforts to Reduce Surgical Wait Times.

Additional funding will allow Ontario to perform thousands more surgeries, procedures and diagnostic imaging hours.

At the height of the third Covid-19 wave in April 2021, all Ontario hospitals were directed to temporarily pause non-urgent clinical activity to preserve capacity to respond to Covid-19 patients.

The government took action to preserve access to urgent surgeries during the pandemic, such as funding support for weekend and evening surgeries. Over 465,000 surgeries took place in main operating rooms in Ontario's hospitals in 2020-2021.

As part of Ontario's 2.5 billion dollar fall preparedness plan, the government has invested 283 million dollars to support additional priority surgeries and procedures, and 457 million dollars to increase community capacity, including home and community care, and to help build more capacity in the health care system to effectively manage the pandemic in the province.

Under the 2021 Budget, Ontario is investing an additional 1.8 billion dollars in the hospital sector in 2021-2022, bringing the total additional investment in hospitals since the start of the pandemic to over 5 billion dollars. This includes temporarily adding more than 3,100 additional hospital beds - the equivalent of six new large community hospitals in the province - to increase capacity and reduce occupancy pressures caused by Covid-19. Many of these beds were used during the pandemic and will continue to be used as part of the province's health care system recovery until at least March 2022.

Ontario's surgical recovery plan will improve the pre- and post-hospital experience for patients by building on ongoing partnerships with Ontario Health Teams and efforts, such as the Digital First for Health strategy and home and community care modernization, with innovative solutions, including centralized surgical waitlist management and funding for home care and transitional care."

I prepared an update for the JET and sent it to the members.

Minutes and Action Log for all PFAC meetings are available. Does the JET wish to receive copies?

Confidentiality Statements have been signed by all PFAC members.

One of the PFAC members, who has been a member of the PFAC since May, has stepped down permanently due to health reasons. The current number of patient, caregiver and family advisors is 3, including me.

Two Working Groups (Clinical Care Redesign and Palliative Care) have scheduled meetings with the PFAC. All PFAC members viewed the overviews of three Working Groups (Retirement Homes, Long Term Care, and Primary Care) provided via video. We need to schedule Digital Health and the Evaluation working groups before the end of September. Project priorities will be established by early October.

We need to finalize the latest article for local papers and social media to increase awareness and interest in the PFAC.

We need COHT partners to post on their websites to assist with PFAC recruitment. PFAC members prefer interested parties contact PFAC in response to promotion rather than receive referrals from the COHT and JET members. We want unbiased individuals who have recent positive and negative experience with the Health Care System and who are not associated with COHT member organizations. This will allow us to determine what is working and what is not working for patients and their families. We also want individuals who are willing to recommend solutions. It is our expectation, that the COHT will hear the negative experiences and consider implementing the solutions if they do not impact medical and clinical operations.

There is a meeting scheduled with the Indigenous Health Circle (IHC) on September 14 to discuss PFAC recruitment from Indigenous communities. BANAC and RAMA are members of the IHC. I confirmed that it was the JET's decision that I be the sole COHT representative and presenter at the BANAC meeting.

I informed the members that I attended the latest meeting of the Northern Muskoka OHT PFAC Network and was invited to chair the meeting on September 29.

PFAC member's orientation has been completed. Members agreed with the level of detail on the presentation slides, provided that hard copies of the slides are shared. Members suggested that interactive activities be included in orientation presentations for consistency with the COHT Shared Value of "having fun".

The Engagement and Partnering Strategy deadline is September 30. The PFAC will assist with the development of the COHT-directed strategy. It was suggested that the document include the phrase "Living Document" to reflect the fact that not all parties have been involved in its development over the summer.

The deadline for the Patient Declaration of Values has been extended to November 30. PFAC has suggested changes to the current document and postponed its discussion until the Ministry of Health provides a revised Ontario Declaration and instructions. It will need to include input from populations in Couchiching area, including Indigenous and vulnerable members.

The PFAC Terms of Reference has been reviewed and discussed by the PFAC. Concern was raised by the members that the Council is named Advisory and that this appears to conflict with the Ontario Health's mandate that the health system be co-designed. PFAC will suggest a name change to reflect the co-design concept.

PFAC will propose metrics to determine PFAC's impact on the COHT and patient care.

Invitations were received and accepted by the PFAC members to attend the next COHT planning meeting on August 19. The agenda should include a welcome and introductions.

August 9

I attended the JET meeting and reviewed the update I sent out yesterday. I left them with much to think about.

August 11

I received a call from a consultant to discuss the COHT website. It took twenty minutes for me to explain the role and presumed impact of PFAC. I stressed that the government indicated that the revamped health system will be co-designed with the input of patients and families and that the COHT website will aid in that endeavor.

I received a call from the co-chair of the JET. She was angry about the tone of my update and recent correspondence. I reminded her that my previous role was to assist Orillia Soldiers Memorial Hospital and local media organizations in obtaining their Ontario Health Team designation. In that role, I recommended they create a patient and caregiver advisory council as part of their application.

The team accepted my recommendation and asked me to assume the role of Chair so I would be present during the interviews with Health Canada auditors. During the interviews, the auditors were impressed with this approach and Health Canada introduced PFAC as a requirement for all Ontario Health Teams.

Now we have received the OHT designation and moved into the co-design stage of the process, I need to take my role as an advocate for patients, families and caregivers seriously. If the PFAC is not involved at the beginning, system improvements that may impact jobs will not be considered. I said that the change in my correspondence reflects that transition and I apologize if she interpreted my constructive criticism as negativity. I also said they may need to consider a new Chair, one who does not come with the history I have with the COHT. At that point, I ended the call.

I was upset about the conversation and how I ended it. I was disappointed that all the work I had put into the COHT and PFAC was not appreciated and that they did not understand the new role I had been assigned.

The government expected improvements in efficiency, reduction in redundancy and improved transparency. That would not be possible if those whose jobs may be changed or eliminated are the same individuals who are re-designing the system.

August 12

After much thought the previous evening and discussion with my family, this morning I made the decision to step down from my volunteer work with the Ontario Health Team. I have been involved for over three years, and my new role is not what I expected. I now realize that they assumed I would continue to be a supportive COHT team player rather than a patient advocate.

I sent an email to the coordinator and the co-chairs of the JET advising my decision to step down on November 1 as the Chair of PFAC and I offered to help them find a suitable replacement. When I hit the email send button, I felt a huge weight lift off my shoulders. I intend to continue my non-political volunteer work, something that I thoroughly enjoy.

Today, Dr. Tam, Canada's Chief Public Health Officer announced that the fourth wave of the Covid-19 pandemic was underway, driven by the Delta variant, with over 13,000 active cases, more than double two weeks prior.

August 13

The Minister of Intergovernmental Affairs and the Transport Minister announced that the federal government planned to mandate the vaccination of all federal public servants, employees in federally regulated transport industries, and passengers of commercial air travel, interprovincial rail service, and large marine vessels with overnight accommodations (e.g. cruise ships). The government also "expected" the vaccination of all employees in industries regulated by the Canada Labour Code. The Government of Canada estimated that there were approximately 19,000 employers and 1,235,000 employees (eight percent of all workers in Canada) subject to the vaccine mandate.

August 15

The early federal election was confirmed for September 20. It was called just days after the Dr. Tam announced we were in a fourth wave of the pandemic. I find this very irresponsible.

August 16

I called into the JET meeting. Nothing was said about me stepping down, and in fact, there were no questions for me, which was very unusual. So, after the meeting, I sent a courtesy email to the other members of the JET to advise of my plans.

August 17

I chaired the PFAC meeting. I asked the coordinator to introduce the new members to the COHT on Thursday because I will be on the road and not able to actively participate in the meeting. However, I would call in to listen.

During the meeting, the Clinical Care Re-design (CCR) Working Group reviewed their objectives.

One PFAC member will be welcomed to CCR once their work plan has been established. The Chair of the CCR emphasized that the PFAC member must be a good fit, feel comfortable/passionate and meet time requirements.

PFAC should discuss our involvement – we can offer differing perspectives of the health care system.

The work plan will be brought to PFAC for review and input as a group.

It was acknowledged that Ministry driven items must be accomplished.

They need to ensure disclosure if a relationship exists between the patient and one of the member organizations.

The Ontario Chief Medical Officer issued a directive requiring hospitals and home and community care providers to create a policy demanding proof of full vaccination, a valid medical exemption or completion of an education session.

I finalized an article for distribution to reporters and I considered it my last contribution to the Health Team.

Community Update - Couchiching Ontario Health Team

Over two years ago, the Ontario Government introduced a new concept for *integrated health care* and *enhanced system navigation*. This new model of care was introduced as “Ontario Health Teams”, with the overall goal of working with patients, families and service providers to co-design an integrated health care system, allowing for easier system navigation and enhanced transitions between providers.

With a positive reputation for collaborative working relationships, the Couchiching region was successful in establishing one of the first OHTs in the Province; now known as the “Couchiching Ontario Health Team”. The Couchiching Ontario Health Team (Couchiching OHT) is comprised of over twenty organizations spread throughout Orillia, Oro-Medonte, Ramara, Severn and Rama First Nations. These committed organizations are working together to improve patient outcomes by coordinating all aspects of health promotion, disease prevention and integrated care as a unified Team.

As we progressively emerge out of the Covid-19 pandemic, we are able to redirect efforts back to enhancing the concept of seamless, integrated care for our region. For patients, families and care givers, this will mean easier access to services, more effective communication amongst providers and enhanced health outcomes.

The transition in the overall health system to a team-based model, does require time to allow for system transformation to occur. The Couchiching OHT has been working diligently throughout the pandemic to facilitate services such as Covid-19 testing, vaccination, virtual care and will continue to develop this innovative model of care to address the needs of our community.

The following Question and Answer section aims to provide additional information on how the Couchiching OHT is progressing.

Who are the Couchiching OHT members?

The Couchiching OHT is comprised of a variety of core partners and affiliate support members. Our overall membership includes representation from: acute care, primary care, palliative care, home and community care, long-term care, retirement homes, community support services, paramedicine, mental health and addictions, varying levels of government, indigenous service partners and more.

What is the Purpose of the Couchiching OHT?

One of the first steps in the formation of the Couchiching OHT was to create a shared purpose amongst our partner organizations. With feedback from many organizational leaders, staff, patients and caregivers the following shared purpose statement was created:

We are one community that is committed to improving health and wellbeing. Together, we will achieve our goal through system co-design in a culturally safe and meaningful way.

There are several important elements to our shared purpose. We are committed to improving health, not just treating illness alone. Taking a holistic approach to all aspects of wellbeing is critical. The Couchiching OHT will co-design the system with patients, clients, families and caregivers in a way that makes sense to those who need the services. We value relationships and inclusivity, building off the strengths of our partners. The Indigenous saying, "Mitakuye-Oyasin" translated as "all my relations", reflects how we are all connected.

What are some of the examples of the work done to date?

The Couchiching OHT has identified several key areas of focus although there are efforts underway to integrate care for a number of populations. We are committed to engaging our community as this work evolves.

Supporting Our Vulnerable Communities

The Couchiching OHT, Social Determinants of Health (SDOH) working group is a very diverse group of social service agencies, local shelters, food bank, community minded individuals, Indigenous health leaders and municipal leaders who meet regularly to address the needs of the most vulnerable in our community. This includes individuals facing housing and food insecurity, inclusive of those suffering with addiction and mental health disorders and any community members or groups in need.

During Covid-19, this group was called upon to provide innovative ways of providing testing and vaccinations to those who might not otherwise have access. Innovative ideas and partnerships between agencies arose to enhance outreach services and temporary "pop-up" clinics to address the need for outreach-based testing and vaccination.

The SDOH working group continues to provide leadership and remains committed to supporting the new medical centre at the

Lighthouse with patient and programming support, advocating and applying for any additional funding for affordable housing and pursuing a more integrated local system for mental health and addiction care services.

What are some of the key priorities going forward?

The Couchiching OHT is focused on improving health service challenges that face patients, families and caregivers. Recognizing that navigation of the complex healthcare system can be overwhelming for individuals, the Couchiching OHT aims to create fewer, seamless points of entry for people to access and navigate care.

Enhancing communication between providers is also an important goal of all Ontario Health Teams. Currently, an individual's health record is not easily shared between providers, requiring additional work for patients and their providers to share important information. Having a single, comprehensive care plan that can be access by patients, caregivers and providers will be an important step forward to enhancing patient care and communication.

How can you participate as a patient, family or caregiver?

Creating an integrated health care system requires significant change in the way we look at health and wellness in our community. Our goal is to transform our system with patients, families and caregivers as partners.

The Couchiching OHT has formed a Patient and Family Advisory Council (PFAC) to determine the needs of residents in Orillia, Oro-Medonte, Severn, Ramara and Rama First Nations. The purpose of the PFAC is to make recommendations on matters that impact the experience of patients, caregivers and families, and to work with the Couchiching OHT to shape and redesign seamless healthcare services to meet the needs of the Couchiching area. The role of the PFAC is to advance patient engagement and patient-centered care in all services provided by the Couchiching OHT, provide a forum for patients, caregivers and families to identify opportunities to improve the quality of care and to promote opportunities for collaboration among patients, caregivers, families and members of the Couchiching OHT.

The PFAC is a group of volunteers who are not part of the health care system who are seeking members from the community to ensure a diverse and inclusive advisory council. Members are not required to have a background in health care, rather volunteers should be a patient, family member or caregiver who has accessed healthcare services in the Couchiching area during the past five years.

August 18

PM Trudeau stated that “unvaccinated people (with or without medical exemptions) would not be able to board planes or trains in Canada.” He made this statement during a federal election campaign stop in Vancouver, responding to a question about accommodations for unvaccinated travelers.

Our son’s father-in-law and I had a heated discussion about the mRNA Covid-19 vaccine. He was angry and accused me of talking his daughter and her family against receiving the vaccine. I explained that I merely provided the information they had requested and that they made their own decision. He said that he and his wife would have died of Covid-19 if they had not taken the shot and that the vaccine would bring the pandemic to an end if everyone did their part and got the shot. He added that I didn’t know what I was talking about.

I had heard that he and his wife received both doses and were very sick after each of the shots and that his sister-in-law died of cardiac arrest two weeks after receiving her second dose of vaccine. However, I did not react to his insult, one I had heard several times during the pandemic, in fear that I would say something I may regret. What I wanted to say was that he, like so many others, put too much faith in the politicians.

August 19

One of the main agenda items for today's JET meeting was the correspondence I sent to the JET, including patient involvement and the community updates.

August 23

I prepared and recorded the news.

"Ontario reported 650 new cases of Covid-19 on Friday, 689 on Saturday and 722 on Sunday, the highest number since June.

In response to evolving data around the Delta variant and based on the recent experiences of other jurisdictions, the government, in consultation with Ontario's Chief Medical Officer of Health, is pausing the exit from the Roadmap to Reopen.

The Chief Medical Officer of Health and other health experts will continue to monitor the data to determine when it is safe to exit the Roadmap and lift most of the public health and workplace safety measures currently in place."

I participated in the JET meeting. I found it very irritating and tried to hide my emotions during the meeting, but I was not very successful.

September 7 is the deadline for hospital staff to submit their Covid-

19 vaccination status. The hospital decided to require full vaccination status without an exemption, resulting in terminations for non-compliance. I made a comment that coercing someone to receive an experimental drug was unethical. I also mentioned that the government allowed medical exemptions or completion of an education session as is the policy for influenza vaccination.

I was told that the hospital has the legal right to protect other staff members and patients by ensuring that all staff are vaccinated. I responded that may be the case but there is no evidence that the vaccine stops infection or spread and that PPE is worn by all staff in contact with patients.

I wondered out loud what the union's position was on this stance and why they did not protect the rights of their members. I was not surprised when there was nothing but silence in response to my comments.

During my presentation, I informed the JET that I participated in a Northern PFAC Network meeting as did two other JET members. Two of the contentious topics during that meeting were compensation and COHT oversight. It was the consensus of the PFAC members that patient and caregiver input is as important as medical input. Therefore, reimbursement for patients' out-of-pocket expenses is essential to ensure fairness.

It was also the consensus of the network that COHT attendance at

PFAC meetings should be by invitation only. For example, if clarification of current procedures or limitations is desirable as part of the PFAC's review. The PFAC should be autonomous and free to discuss sensitive issues. There was total disagreement expressed by the JET members, so I reminded them of the Purpose and Role of the PFAC as approved by the JET.

PURPOSE

Determine the needs of residents in Orillia, Oro-Medonte, Severn, Ramara and Rama.

Make recommendations on matters that impact the experience of patients and families.

Work with COHT to shape and redesign seamless healthcare services to meet the needs of the area.

ROLE

Advise COHT on meeting the needs of patients, caregivers and families.

Advance patient engagement and patient-centered care in all services provided by COHT.

Provide a forum for patients, caregivers and families to identify opportunities to improve matters impacting the experience of patients, caregivers and families.

Promote opportunities for collaboration among patients, caregivers, families and members of COHT.

August 25

The Chair of the JET called me at 7:00 am to discuss the last JET meeting and the community updates. He graciously thanked me for all the hard work I put in over the past six years. He was especially appreciative of the fact that I am retired and that my advice was not biased by financial gain. He expressed his concern that my relationship with one of the JET members seemed strained as of late and that my attitude had changed. I reminded him that in my role as Chair of the PFAC I now speak for the other members of the PFAC and patients I meet in our community.

After the call, I told my husband that I thought the Chair was very condescending and his goal was to silence me. I see no reason not to support the hospital staff who were regarded as heroes just a few months ago. I also see no reason to withhold crucial information about the vaccine that they are recommending to their staff.

I enrolled in multiple Indigenous Culture courses scheduled from September through November. I sent an email to BANAC Health Circle reminding them about the meeting September 14 and to let them know that I had registered for the courses.

August 27

I spoke to our next-door neighbor about the Victorian Order of

Nurses (VON) adult daycare, and he gave me contact information. He takes his wife two times each week to give him a break. I called my friend with the information so she can enroll her adult son with special needs into the program.

August 30

The JET meetings for today and Monday were cancelled presumably due to the long weekend.

August 31

I chaired the PFAC meeting.

I agreed to send my news articles to the members.

The JET retreat was discussed, and it was agreed that I will bring feedback to the PFAC members after the meeting.

A survey will go to patients and caregivers in general and to frail seniors with a coordinated care plan. The results of the two groups will be compared. We will plan a follow-up survey based on the results.

In preparation for the next Northern PFAC Network meeting, our members will propose agenda items. Two suggestions I made were -Measurement of success, and

Standardization of PFACs.

I requested input from the members after they have reviewed the slides for the BANAC meeting on September 14.

A Palliative Care presentation is planned for the next PFAC meeting.

I made no mention of the recent JET meeting or my conversation with the Chair after the meeting.

Chapter 20 – SEPTEMBER 2021

September 6

I prepared and recorded the news.

"The province reported 944 new cases of Covid-19 on Saturday and 811 on Sunday.

The Provincial Science Table concluded that reducing contacts and increasing vaccines will help slow the fourth wave.

The doctors watching Covid-19 in Ontario say some intervention – but not necessarily a lockdown – will be needed during the fourth wave to prevent ICUs from being overwhelmed again.

At the current rates of the fourth wave, the Table expects about 500 Covid-19 patients in ICUs by October and predicts ICUs will be "overwhelmed beyond what we saw in the third wave."

The Delta variant has changed the province's Covid-19 response already, prompting the Chief Medical Officer to announce a pause on the Roadmap to Reopening to hold current restrictions in place until further notice.

A report by Public Health Ontario in July stated previous estimates of vaccine coverage needed to begin lifting public health measures were based on the Alpha variant, and should be revised for the Delta variant. The province's Roadmap to Reopen was based on Alpha variant vaccination rates, and stated Ontario could exit the plan with seventy-five per cent of the eligible population vaccinated.

"Because of the Delta variant, and to avoid a lockdown in the fall, vaccination needs to accelerate … and we need to reduce contacts," stated the Science Table press release.

According to the Science Table's last release, the Delta variant has a reproductive number between six and eight, meaning every person infected typically passes the virus on to six-to-eight other people. The original Covid-19 strain had a reproductive number between two and three.

The risk of hospitalization and intensive care admission after infection is also two-to-three times higher with the Delta variant, according to the Science Table.

On Sept. 1 a vaccine passport program was announced requiring people to show proof of vaccination to go indoors at restaurants, gyms, and other public settings.

The Ontario Department of Health previously issued orders for high-risk settings to implement vaccination policies, which includes colleges and universities, shelters, retirement homes, group homes, health care settings, paramedics, and others.

Loved ones reflect on local lives lost to opioid 'epidemic'

Earlier this week, friends and loved ones of those who have died due to a drug overdose, met in downtown Orillia to honour and reflect on the lives lost.

Carolyn Jones, a registered public health nurse with the Simcoe Muskoka District Health Unit, said the event was to mark International Overdose Awareness Day.

"Opioid overdoses have become an epidemic in our world and our country."

Jones says the opioid crisis is becoming a major problem in Orillia, and she says it's time the public becomes more aware and involved to put a stop to it."

I prepared an agenda for the Northern PFAC Network meeting that I will chair and sent it to the members.

I sent an email to the COHT coordinator about the Ontario Health PFAC Engagement Strategy. I provided several comments from the members of the PFAC.

Our son called and asked me to send him links to Health Canada websites that provide copies of the Emergency Release Regulations, the Vaccine and Gene Therapy regulations, summaries of data that supported each of the Covid-19 vaccine releases, and the Product Monographs for each of the vaccines. His wife wanted to review these documents in preparation for a conversation she planned to have with her parents. She is worried about her parents getting more vaccine shots and wants to convince them that the vaccine is not safe for everyone and may cause long-term effects. She also plans to show them that the clinical trials did not examine infection, disease spread or deaths and used a different manufacturing process from the one used for mass injection. The trials only looked at hospitalization in vaccinated versus unvaccinated over a period of three months. All the information on the website I provided was public. Anyone with any interest can access the information required to make an informed decision.

September 7

The hospital vaccine mandate takes effect today. I heard from one of the staff that they were given their notice. It is so upsetting for them and their family, especially considering that she had Covid-19 early in the pandemic and risked her life to save others. I said that she may be better off looking for a change in career, one which will allow her to work from home. My heart breaks for her and others all across Canada who are in the same situation. They took the time to access the risks and benefits, made the best decision for them and their families, and are now being punished for it.

The situation between our daughter-in-law and her parents is not good. They refuse to listen to reason and continue to accuse her of being selfish for not getting vaccinated. This argument is an echo of similar sentiments expressed by the government and news channels all across Canada. There has even been talk in a Toronto newspaper and on popular news programs about denying unvaccinated people emergency medical treatment.

September 10

We went to the advanced Federal Election voting station this morning. We were made to line up outside in the rain keeping our masks on and a distance of two meters. We were soaked by the time we got inside. Once there, we were greeted by an individual behind a Plexi-glass screen. She came around the screen to hand us the ballot and a pencil. She told us to complete the card, place the ballot into the box and then throw away the pencil before exiting the building by the back door. I do not understand how they expect these procedures to stop an airborne virus from spreading. The only thing that these measures accomplished was wasting taxpayers' money.

September 12

I received a meeting link and an agenda from the BANAC Health Circle for the conference call on September fourteenth.

Prior to the upcoming JET meeting, I received the following information and a script to be read by administration staff when calling unvaccinated individuals. This is part of a government initiative to increase vaccine uptake. I forwarded the information to the PFAC members and requested their input.

Starting late this week, the Provincial Vaccine Contact Centre (PVCC) will begin conducting outbound calls to the approximately 720,000 unvaccinated, unrostered adults across Ontario. The PVCC will be reaching out to these individuals to:

Encourage them to get their vaccine.

Provide information about how the Delta variant continues to be a risk.

Provide information about the upcoming proof of vaccination requirement in prescribed settings as of September 22, 2021.

Book an appointment if the individual is amenable (or provide information on how they may book an appointment locally or access other channels such as pharmacy, mobile clinics, etc.)

The script included claims that the Covid-19 vaccines are safe for everyone, including pregnant women, lactating women, women who plan to get pregnant within the next few months and people with autoimmune conditions. These claims contradict the information in the manufacturers' product information brochures.

Effective 12:01 a.m. on September 22, 2021, Ontario will require patrons to provide proof of identification and Covid-19 vaccination to access certain businesses and settings. A FAQ document was released to provide more specific information to the public and businesses about this program.

Between September 22 and October 22, 2021, in addition to proof of identity, a patron must show a paper or digital version of the PDF receipt of their proof of vaccination or their proof of valid medical exemption from their doctor or nurse practitioner.

The province is developing a digital version of the enhanced vaccine certificate with QR code that people will use to gain access to designated settings that will be launched on October 22nd. Paper copies of the PDF receipt will also continue to be an option as well.

People who have a green and white health card can access their proof of vaccination through the Ontario provincial booking portal, or by calling the Provincial Vaccine Contact Centre. People with red and white health cards can call the Provincial Vaccine Contact Centre to have their receipt emailed to them. Individuals who do not have a health card can contact the health unit to verify their identity and have a Covid-19 ID/Personal Access Code issued. Individuals can then call the Provincial Vaccine Contact Centre to provide this Covid-19 ID to arrange to receive their vaccine receipt by email.

I received several comments from the PFAC members expressing concern about patient confidentiality and the potential of spreading false information by the individuals making the calls. I forwarded the comments to the JET.

September 13

I prepared and recorded the news.

“The province reported 857 new cases of Covid-19 on Saturday and 784 on Sunday. Restrictions remain in place including mandatory vaccination for high-risk indoor settings such as restaurants and bars. Vaccine passports will be issued by Ontario for use by vaccinated individuals to allow them into restricted areas. Many companies are refusing to mandate vaccination due to the threat of legal suits by employees and others are refusing to discriminate against those who have not been vaccinated. Wearing a mask and social distancing remains the best practice when going out in public.

'Ousted' students had their connection to school severed when learning first moved online since they had limited or no access to the internet at home.

Students who have fallen out of the education system due to the pandemic, risk diminished prospects, and the Ontario government needs a major outreach effort to bring missing students back to its classrooms, says the head of a global commission for education recovery.

Ontario's education response to Covid-19 has led to a significant number of students slipping through the cracks.

In the initial days and weeks of the pandemic, schools around the world responded in mostly the same way, closing immediately upon recording a case of the virus. But as time went on, some education systems stayed shut longer than others or closed quicker when cases spiked.

Ontario shut down in-person learning for 28 weeks between March 2020 and summer 2021, the longest collection of system-wide school closures in Canada pivoting to remote virtual instruction while schools were shuttered.

Statistics Canada data on households with children found 1.2 per cent did not have access to the internet at home prior to the pandemic. Households with less income were much more likely to be unconnected.

Those unable to get online were likely joined by students living in abusive situations, as well as children in new immigrant homes with limited or no English or French, those feeling labour pressures that may have grown over time for families struggling through the pandemic, and children in Indigenous communities.

Teens who have lost interest in school or were unable to access virtual learning at home during the school closures may have gone into the work force, into the streets, into gangs or begin self-destructive behaviour.

Ontario's current plan for schools is "designed to minimize disruption and maximize safety," including by requiring staff to be fully vaccinated or get tested weekly and investing in improvements to ventilation. The province has not said what specific thresholds or metrics would spark a school closure in the upcoming school year.

The province is also making easier Covid-19 testing options available — including take-home tests for many high school students — in a bid to reduce absenteeism Annie Kidder, executive director of People for Education, said safety was an important consideration for Ontario's two million school-age children, but that they also need mental health and learning supports in an equitable, welcoming place that prepares them for the future.

At the JET meeting today, I reviewed the PFAC’s comments and concerns, specifically the breaking of confidentiality by sharing names and phone numbers of individuals who have not been vaccinated and the unsupported claims that the vaccine is safe in untested populations. I was attacked again by the same member of the team who attacked me previously. She accused me of not educating the PFAC members and making negative comments during JET meetings. I expressed my surprise and confusion, clarified my role as Chair of the PFAC and suggested that the interaction between the JET and PFAC needs to be reviewed.

I was disappointed that the coordinator, who attends all PFAC meetings, did not come to my defense. However, I understood, that if he spoke up, his contract position may be put into jeopardy. After the meeting I sent an email to the coordinator about the approach to the PFAC meeting scheduled for tomorrow.

September 14

This is shaping up to be a very busy day.

It started with a PFAC meeting at 10:00 am.

The Palliative Care Working Group made a presentation and then left the meeting.

I reviewed the JET's response to the PFAC comments regarding the outreach initiative and script.

We discussed the Engagement Strategy.

We reviewed the public's awareness and understanding of palliative care and when to ask for it.

There are few if any palliative care doctors in the area.

We reviewed the news article about the COHT and PFAC.

We discussed the planned patient surveys.

As requested by the JET, I participated in a Health System Performance Network conference call at 12:00 pm. They reviewed Health Equity, a patient experience question after every visit with a practitioner and a Best Practices Tool Kit. It was agreed that these meetings will occur the first Tuesday of every month. I sent an email to the JET recommending that they assign a member to join the

HSPN meetings with me.

I made my presentation to the BANAC Health Circle at 1:30 pm. There were no questions after the presentation other than a request to obtain a copy of the slides. The Chair of the Circle then explained why they would NOT join the COHT or PFAC.

The Health Circle are proceeding with an Indigenous OHT. They are currently at the self-assessment stage. No Indigenous OHT has been approved by the government, and they will not receive funding without a OHT designation. They will send me the Position Statement for an OHT Indigenous Engagement in Simcoe Muskoka after the meeting. I offered to be available to help with their application or provide contact information for other COHT members to discuss OHT application issues.

In summary, my presentation to the BANAC Indigenous Health Circle was received respectfully. However, the response in the end was that participation on our PFAC only made sense if they were equal partners on the COHT. Concern was expressed by members that if they joined the COHT, they would be relinquishing their ability to self-govern and to control their own health services. They are planning to submit their own Indigenous Ontario Health Team application in the near future. Partnerships may be available once approval has been received by Ontario Health.

It was stated that any member of their community is free to provide advice to our PFAC and my contact information will be made available to their community members.

I provided an update to the JET and advised them of the BANAC's final decision.

September 15

No meetings today. However, I received an email from the Administrative Assistant of the JET that I will need to have two doses of Covid-19 vaccine, with the last received at least two weeks before the meeting, to attend the COHT Retreat on September 23. This information was not provided previously, and I had informed the JET that I do not intend to get the shot. My position has been that I am not an employee, so mandates do not apply to me.

I immediately sent the following email to the other two members of the PFAC

The JET has planned an all-day RETREAT for next Thursday September 23.

I am unable to attend. Are either of you able and willing to attend? The details are below. You must be fully vaccinated at least 14 days in advance.

One of the members, who is also retired, called me and said she had not received the vaccine so will be unable to attend.

The other member sent me an email and said she may be able to attend IF she can get the day off work. She followed up with an email one hour later and said she will attend in place of me.

I immediately sent an email to the Administrative Assistant to let her know that I could not attend, provided my reason and relayed the name of my substitute.

Within minutes I received the following email from the same person who continues to attack me.

“My Administrator has just advised me that you are unable to attend our OHT retreat due to the new provincial rules around Covid-19 vaccination proof that will be required which goes into effect next week.

This is an important planning day and the voice and presence of a PFAC member is key so I would ask if you could please send a delegate in your place. Kindly advise them that all out of pocket expenses will be covered for the day.

If you could let me know who will be representing the PFAC, I'd appreciate that.”

I forwarded the email to her that I had sent to the Admin. There was no reply. I should have pointed out that the provincial rules allow medical exemptions. However, the medical community has chosen more stringent requirements. I bit my tongue and left it well enough alone. My long and successful career taught me that I must choose my battles carefully.

September 16

This Covid-19 pandemic has brought the worst out in some people and the best in others. So many of my family and friends are having relationship problems. Marriages have been destroyed, friendships ended, brother and sisters not talking, parents and adult children arguing and grandchildren missing family gatherings. It makes me so angry when world leaders do not consider the damage to society or the economy when they make policies which are not helpful in stopping the pandemic.

My husband and I are volunteers at the Repair Café tomorrow. We will try to fix broken items people bring to the café. We spent a few hours packing the tools and supplies we may need. This is the third time we have been involved. It makes us feel good to see things given a second life.

I sent the new Patient Family Caregiver Declaration of Values to the PFAC members for review and comment.

September 18

We arrived at the Café, which was held in our shopping mall this year due to the Covid-19 restrictions. Fortunately, the proof of vaccination requirements will not be in effect until next week.

Before we opened for business, the organizers gave us packages of wet wipes to use on our hands. I noticed right away that they contain hydrogen chloride (bleach) which can damage skin. Those wipes are for the decontamination of surfaces only. I informed everyone not to use them and that they should only use wipes containing alcohol. This made me think about how little medical knowledge the public possesses and why politicians can convince them to do things that are not in their best interest.

Individuals were staged in a separate area and came to our table one at a time. Everyone was wearing masks. When we completed the repair, the customer left by one door and the new customer came by another entrance.

One of the most interesting items we repaired was a life-sized animated Santa Claus. The next day we saw a picture of us standing next to the Santa posted in our local paper.

September 20

It is Federal Election Day.

I prepared and recorded the news.

"The province reported 821 new cases of Covid-19 on Saturday and 715 on Sunday. Restrictions remain in place including mandatory vaccination for high-risk indoor settings such as restaurants and bars. Vaccine passports will be required after Sept 22 to allow vaccinated individuals into restricted areas. Wearing a mask and social distancing whether fully vaccinated or not remain the best practices when going out in public and are recommended by the W.H.O. and Health Canada. Studies demonstrate that for the prevention of spread of Covid-19 variants, surgical masks are more effective than cloth.

New local cannabis store targets 'those who are suffering'

Orillia's only independent and locally owned cannabis store is taking a unique approach aimed at helping people who are suffering.

Vivid Cannabis Co. store manager says her store boasts a first-responder program to help pave the way for people with physical and mental health concerns to get support.

Vivid is working on developing a lab where they will plan to launch Orillia's first farm-gate production site store which would allow customers to purchase cannabis products directly from the producer.

Vivid's location is close to OPP Headquarters and Orillia Soldiers' Memorial Hospital (OSMH).

Council to get update on future hospital plans, Age-Friendly Orillia

Today is federal election day, but it's also city council day.

Prior to the 4:00 p.m. council meeting, a public meeting will take place at 1:00 p.m. regarding a request for a zoning bylaw amendment that would potentially pave the way for a new veterinarian clinic.

The virtual council meeting will begin with an update on the future hospital project.

Up next will be an update on the Age-Friendly Community Needs Assessment and Action Plan.

Online and telephone voting in the next municipal election will be back before council members at today's meeting.

In August, council committee voted against a staff recommendation that called for internet and telephone voting. It was decided the matter would come to council for possible ratification today to allow time for public feedback on potential voting methods.

Volunteers work to keep items out of landfill

A free Repair Café, hosted by Sustainable Orillia as part of Sustainable Orillia Month at Orillia Square mall, was busy Saturday.

The event gave people an opportunity to see if local tech junkies and avid do-it-yourselfers could fix appliances and household items to keep them from unnecessarily clogging up Orillia's landfill.

The goal of the Repair Café is to extend the life of many products through the community helping each other out and lending a hand.

On Saturday, volunteers were on hand to sew and mend clothes, fix computers, cellphones and small electrical appliances, repair jewellery, assist with woodworking, among other things.

Thirty-three items were brought in for repair, twenty-five of them were fixed resulting in one hundred and thirty kilograms diverted from the landfill."

The President of the Hospital, the Clinical Care Manager, the PFAC Coordinator and the Administrative Assistant all asked for my help with documents today. I am looking forward to removing myself from this obligation after November 1.

September 21

We are in for another four years of the Trudeau Liberals as a minority government.

I met with the two other PFAC members this morning and told them about my plans to step down. The meeting was productive although neither want to be the Chair due to the heavy workload. I tried to convince them that much of the work I do for the COHT is an overflow of the volunteer history I have with the hospital and COHT before I became Chair of the PFAC. The new chair will not be asked to contribute to as many initiatives. They said that they now understand why I behave more like a COHT member than a patient advisor. I agreed and said that is why I am stepping down as Chair. I suggested that they should consider co-chairing the PFAC.

The Administrator asked for help with updates needed for the Retreat. I completed several documents, that included the update I sent to the JET on September 14 and sent them to her.

The Coordinator of the COHT sent me an invitation to a video conference tomorrow at 9:00 am.

September 22

During the meeting with the coordinator, we discussed the Patient Engagement Strategy, PFAC reimbursement, and PFAC meeting scheduling. I explained that for the past three years, as a volunteer, I did not receive any compensation for the many hours spent working with the hospital and COHT committees. That was not an issue for me because I am retired and do not need the money to pay my bills. If future volunteers are still working and the COHT needs the meetings to be held during normal work hours, volunteer PFAC members should receive compensation to make up for lost pay or vacation time. If the meetings are held on weekends or weekday evenings, only out of pocket expenses need to be paid to the volunteers. Salaried medical staff are expected to work after hours, and they receive reimbursement for out-of-pocket expenses. It is a matter of equity and fairness for all. He asked me to put that in writing to the JET, which I did after the call -

This recommendation to the JET is from the PFAC members.

To minimize barriers and to ensure patient, family and caregiver participation in the co-design of the COHT health care system, the following options are presented for consideration:

1. Hold meetings during evenings or weekends to allow patients, family and caregivers to participate, or

2. Hold meetings during work hours in the week and reimburse patients, family and caregivers for loss of salary.

It is understood that members and partners of the COHT and JET are not at a financial disadvantage when attending COHT and JET meetings.

Thank you in advance for your support.

September 23

I spent a few minutes summarizing the Covid-19 facts in preparation for possible attacks by the JET.

Covid-19 is an airborne virus and is spread by close contact with a contagious individual or in a crowded room for an extended period of time with a contagious individual.

Cloth masks are not effective in stopping a virus from spreading. Surgical masks help reduce transmission by an infected person but do not help the wearer. N95 masks help protect both the wearer and close contacts.

Covid-19 vaccine may reduce the severity of disease.

There is no data to support long-term safety of the vaccines for mass injection.

Vaccinated individuals can be infected and transmit disease.

Unvaccinated individuals are not protected by the vaccinated.

Unvaccinated individuals do not put the vaccinated at risk.

Natural immunity may last longer and be more effective than immunity by mRNA vaccines.

Herd immunity may reduce spread.

Limiting indoor activities may reduce spread.

The only thing that can protect both vaccinated and unvaccinated alike is self-isolation when sick.

September 27

I prepared and recorded the news.

"The province reported 640 new cases of Covid-19 on Saturday and 653 on Sunday. Restrictions remain in place including mandatory vaccination for high-risk indoor settings such as restaurants and bars. Proof of vaccination and identity are now required to allow vaccinated individuals into restricted areas. Vaccine passports will not be available for a few more weeks. The number of vaccinated people allowed in certain settings has increased. Wearing a mask and social distancing whether fully vaccinated or not remain the best practices when going out in public and are recommended by the W.H.O. and Health Canada.

The Simcoe Muskoka District Health Unit is beginning a phased reopening of routine publicly funded child and adult immunization services that were paused in March 2020, due to the increased demands of the Covid-19 pandemic.

Beginning the week of September 27, the health unit will offer public immunization clinics at each of its seven local health unit offices across the region, starting with appointments for those zero to six years of age who are overdue for their routine immunizations. Appointments for adolescent boosters and adult vaccinations will become available in the following weeks. The public is encouraged to continue to check the health unit website for updates as appointments for these groups are added to the schedule.

The health unit is also working with school board partners to resume the Grade seven school immunization program where students are offered Hepatitis B, Meningitis C-ACYW and Human Papillomavirus vaccines at school-based clinics. Those in Grade seven and eight will be offered their vaccines this school year at school-based clinics.

Public immunization clinics are appointment only and can be booked through the health unit's online booking system.

Ontario's dentists regard dental care as health care. With that in mind, the Ontario Dental Association (ODA) said it will provide dental care to all Ontario residents, regardless of their vaccination status.

In a news release issued Wednesday, the ODA said it wanted to clarify some misunderstandings that have come up.

One is that dentists are not allowed to reveal the vaccination status of their employees, such as dental hygienists. That is personal information that is protected by the Personal Health Information Protection Act, said the ODA.

At the same time, the ODA said that Ontario dentists have been leaders in terms of having strict infection prevention procedures so that everyone could get safe dental care despite the pandemic.

Just as important is the fact that the ODA is on record as endorsing, and encouraging, all health care workers to be vaccinated.

"Back in January, the ODA also pushed to get dentists, hygienists and dental staff early access to vaccines," said a statement from ODA communications specialist Maggie Blood.

Patients can rest assured all safety precautions are being taken to keep them protected throughout their appointment, said the ODA statement.

Also, throughout the pandemic, no known cases of Covid-19 have been linked to treatment at an Ontario dental office thanks to all the infection prevention standards in place."

I commend the ODA for their logical approach to the pandemic. The ODA is a model to be admired and practiced. If they can avoid infection and spread, when working close to the inside of the patient's mouth and nose, anyone should be able to do the same. They also observe confidentiality and respect for autonomy. I had hoped that the medical community would have taken the same logical and practical approach during the pandemic. Rather they attacked anyone who disagreed with their policies.

I attended a JET meeting where we discussed the latest update I sent to them a few days before. There were no decisions made during the meeting.

PFAC Update for 27 September 2021

Prepared by Susan Langlois, CHAIR PFAC

- Minutes and Action Logs for all PFAC meetings are available.
- Two Working Groups (Clinical Care Redesign and Palliative Care) have met with the PFAC members. All PFAC members viewed the overviews of three Working Groups (Retirement Homes, Long Term Care, and Primary Care) provided via video by the Chairs. **Need to schedule Digital Health and the Evaluation working groups before the end of**

September. PFAC members will be assigned to Working Groups by the end September.

- Susan met with the BANAC Indigenous Health Circle (IHC) on September 14 to discuss PFAC recruitment from Indigenous communities. BANAC and RAMA are members of the IHC.
- Susan's presentation (copy of slide deck on file with the JET) to the BANAC Indigenous Health Circle on September 14 was received respectfully and a few questions were asked. However, the response in the end was that participation on our PFAC only made sense if they were equal partners on the COHT. Concern was expressed by BANAC members that if they joined the COHT, they would be relinquishing their ability to self-govern and to control their own health services. **They are planning to submit their own Indigenous Ontario Health Team application in the near future. Partnerships may be available once approval has been received by Ontario Health.**
- The IHC provided a copy of their Position Statement to the Ontario Health Teams titled Indigenous Engagement in Simcoe Muskoka (copy on file with the JET).
- The meeting ended with a declaration that any member of the Indigenous community is free to provide advice to our

PFAC and Susan's contact information will be made available to their community members.

- Susan attended the last meeting of the Northern Muskoka OHT PFAC Network and will chair the next meeting on September 29. Topics to be covered are Patient, Family and Caregiver Partnership and Engagement Strategies; Patient, Family and Declaration of Values; Current PFAC activities; Future PFAC plans.
- **The COHT-directed Engagement and Partnering Strategy deadline is September 30. A final review by the PFAC members should be done prior to submission.**
- The PFAC Terms of Reference have been reviewed and discussed by the PFAC. Concern was raised by the members that the Council is named Advisory and that this appears to conflict with the Ontario Health's mandate that the health system be co-designed. **PFAC members suggested that the name be changed to reflect the co-design concept. This would also distinguish the nature of the PFAC partnerships of the past and provide opportunities to reframe the engagement. It was also suggested the Ontario Health should consider a name change. There are precedents for the adoption of a different name for a regional organization, e.g. "Children's Aid" in Orillia**

has been re-named "Family Connections" to better reflect their mandate.

- PFAC will propose metrics to determine PFAC's impact on the COHT and patient care.
- **The deadline for the Patient Declaration of Values has been extended to November 30. The Ministry of Health provided a revised Ontario Declaration in September. A review will be conducted by the PFAC, and recommendations will be made to the JET by the end of September. It should also include input from populations in Couchiching area, including Indigenous and vulnerable members.**
- The two new PFAC members attended the last COHT Collaboration Table meeting on August 19 and one of the new members attended the JET retreat.
- **The following recommendation was sent to the JET from the PFAC members.**
- To minimize barriers and to ensure patient, family and caregiver participation in the co-design of the COHT health care system and participation in Working Group meetings, the following options are presented for consideration:

- Hold meetings during evenings or weekends to allow patients, family and caregivers to participate, or
- Hold meetings during work hours in the week and reimburse patients, family and caregivers for loss of salary in addition to out-of-pocket expenses.

- It is understood that members and partners of the COHT and JET are not at a financial disadvantage when attending COHT and JET meetings during weekdays.

- **The term of the current PFAC Chair expires on November 1, 2021. Susan is not seeking re-election but will stay on to assist with the transition.**

September 28

The day began with a PFAC meeting. Several new issues were discussed and documented.

Meeting Frequency was discussed and all agreed that they should occur monthly, during lunch hour or after hours/end of day. The frequency may be increased if information needs to be discussed or voted on. We will utilize other forms of communication such as voting by email. New members may drive future meeting times. If the Administrator cannot attend, PFAC members will rotate minute taking and only meet when necessary.

The Declaration of Values will be reviewed by members, and suggestions will be submitted to Susan by mid-October.

A Network PFAC meeting is scheduled for September 29th. Susan will chair the meeting and our PFAC members will attend. We will discuss compensation, recruitment (what works), and the current state.

The PFAC Chair position will be vacant as of November 1st. We need a JET discussion regarding transition. The Chair feels all PFAC members should be present at this meeting.

Working groups are at different stages of development. PFAC members are ready and waiting for invitation from working group leads. Susan will attend Long Term Care and Retirement Home working groups. The other PFAC members will decide who would like to participate on the Clinical Care Redesign, Palliative Care and Primary Care working groups.

PFAC will request to add a "suggestion box" on the COHT website. It would be a forum for the public to provide input regarding their experiences within the system and to provide potential solutions.

We require JET support to increase membership, compensation, and involvement with working groups.

After the meeting, I received a Zoom call from the President of the hospital and his assistant. I was surprised by the call. He has never called me by Zoom before. He only used the phone when he needed to speak to me.

He opened the meeting by asking how my meeting with the BANAC Health Circle was received. I told him that they listened respectfully to my presentation, which was approved by the JET. It took about thirty minutes to complete. They did not ask any questions during or after my talk. Then the Chair of the Health Circle told me that they were in the process of applying for an Indigenous OHT and will not join the COHT or PFAC. They may partner with us once they obtain approval for their Indigenous OHT and the government financial support.

He asked if they seemed upset and I told him that they did not make any negative comments to me. I asked him why he was asking me these questions. He said that when he spoke to the Chair, she said that the Health Circle members were offended by my comments during the presentation. I was genuinely shocked and told him so. That was the end of the call.

I felt like I had just been thrown under the bus. At the beginning, I had a gut feeling I should not have met with the Indigenous Community alone and I should have listened to my gut. When I asked for a JET or COHT member to join me, no one offered and said that I should conduct the first meeting myself.

This call really upset me. I could not imagine what I said that could make them so angry as to not want to participate in the reinvention of the health care system. **Then it dawned on me.** They had made their decision long before I met with them. As requested, I sent the slides to them in June. My presentation included all the tools required to apply for their own OHT. They also would realize that government funding is only available for approved OHTs. Now they are using me as the reason the Indigenous Community will not work with the OHT. Very clever indeed.

September 29

I reviewed the PFAC strategy comments provided by the JET and sent my additional comments to the coordinator.

I chaired the Northern PFAC Network meeting. One other PFAC member and a JET member attended the meeting. It was a great discussion with very interesting and knowledgeable individuals.

The Patient, Family and Caregiver Partnership and Engagement Strategy was discussed.

All Nations Health Partners have deferred their review to the end of October. They are meeting with current membership and waiting to have a fulsome discussion/engagement with members.

The Nipissing Wellness OHT Collaborative Council reviewed and developed it with Health Partners. It is considered a living document. It was sent to be translated and will be posted on the website tomorrow. There has been discussion around where it should be posted. If collaboratively developed on behalf of the OHT it should fall under the overall vision, not just a PFAC tab.

The Algoma OHT expect the final proofreading to be completed today and then it will be ready for submission and be up on the website tomorrow.

The COHT will complete it by September 30, and it will be posted on their website when the website is ready.

It was suggested that we exchange the documents amongst the group. It was concluded that visiting websites is most effective.

The group agreed that the PFAC role should be to bring system failures to the OHT and propose alternative practices. This requires a wide range of patient experiences from different sections of the system.

The names of most PFACs have been modified to reflect co-design, partnerships and caregivers. The new names will show up on websites, the COHT PFAC is reviewing a potential name change.

The Recruitment process was discussed

One OHT have developed a Communications Committee and

accessed Community Engagement Strategists, created a matrix at the beginning to target who would be needed to have a fulsome group. Social media, print and mailbox stuffing. Door to door mailers is just as effective. Encourage people that completing the application is not necessary, interest is more important than your time and ability to fill it out. Information will be obtained during the interview.

Another OHT asked who isn't here – who do we need to hear from, don't make assumptions based on what people have shared. Building trust, understand skills (skills mapping – chart what you hope to have and offer to membership). Video with Canadore students, used in social media, gatherings, engage students. Expression of Interest: face to face interview to get a sense of who each person is. Who are the networks related to existing OHT partners? Intergenerational gaps. Script working with professor at the college, they will document the process so that others can use it. Healthcare retired members – can have both healthcare side as well as caregiver/patient. Fresh eyes are also helpful. Potential for "interesting dynamic". PFAC first. "Slowly, thoughtfully, respectfully". Must move forward.

A third OHT posted the Expression of Interest on their website (district of Muskoka). Sent out to all partners, social media and an article in the paper. Seventeen to twenty have been interviewed, questions were provided in advance, they now have thirteen PFAC members in total. Age group thirty to eighty. Two people have since stepped down. Onboarding/orientation – participation now in working groups. Retired healthcare workers who are now either patients or caregivers can be gems!

Engagement is next stage, reach out to communities not at the table. Go to them, understand the process – Nation to Nation, visit rural areas.

Retired health care workers bring a unique lens, providing care for family but also understanding the barriers. Interview process could reveal if that person is right for the PFAC. How do you obtain a diverse group when paid staff work 9-5? We need to accommodate, be flexible and utilize digital platforms.

The Patient Declaration of Values was discussed.

A new name was proposed to include Family and Caregiver. It was confirmed that there is no option, we are just adopting and attesting.

Deadline for posting is November 30th. Will need to wait and see if the PFAC comments have flexibility with the adoption.

It was proposed the during the next meeting we should decide when to speak to the Ministry and what message we want to support each other in. The main barrier is tight timelines, deadlines and fast turnaround times. Proper engagement is impossible and is eroding trust. We are set up to fail. Resources and efficiencies are not available when we are already in a deficit. We need to slow down!

The North is ignored. Funding is available but we are unable to access it. We should request a Minister attend a meeting to hear from each Northern OHT.

Much of the meeting reflected the frustration I expressed to the JET over the past year. It was good that one of the JET was present to hear the frustration of other PFAC Chairs. Hopefully, my next discussion with them will not land on deaf ears. The government is using the Ontario Health Team as a campaign success story and claim that the health care system has been co-designed with patients. The pandemic clearly demonstrated that the health system requires major modernization and if it is to be successful, patient voices must be heard and understood. Rushing the process only serves the politicians need to demonstrate progress.

September 30

Today is a National Reconciliation Holiday.

I spent most of my day downloading and reading Indigenous information in preparation for my courses.

Chapter 21 – OCTOBER 2021

October 1

I reviewed the latest version of the COHT Engagement Strategy in preparation for the JET meeting. I noticed that most of my comments were rejected. This is so frustrating. I spent a lot of time on these documents. My comments were positive and in line with other PFAC engagement strategies. I just don't understand what the objections are to taking things more slowly to ensure we obtain various experiences, even if they are negative. We need to learn by our mistakes. That is the only way to improve the system. Status quo is not what we should be striving for.

October 2

I finished reading all the Indigenous documents. I found them very interesting and informative and shared them with the other members of the PFAC.

October 4

We packed the RV and are getting ready for our mini vacation starting tomorrow.

I recorded the news.

The province reported 668 new cases of Covid-19 on Saturday and

580 on Sunday.

Long-term care home staff must be double vaxxed by November 15

Ontario is mandating Covid-19 vaccines for long-term care staff.

The policy is effective November 15. It affects all in-home staff, support workers, students and volunteers unless they have a valid medical exemption.

The province also announced it is expanding inspections of homes and redirecting provincial resources to enhance audit testing in homes.

The new requirements for homes are:

Staff, support workers, students and volunteers must show proof of being fully vaccinated or show proof of a valid medical exemption. A person is considered fully vaccinated fourteen days after receiving their second dose.

Staff who aren't fully vaccinated or have a valid medical exemption won't be able to enter a long-term care home to work.

New hires must be fully vaccinated before starting work.

Homes will randomly test fully vaccinated people, including staff, caregivers and visitors, for possible breakthrough cases.

The province doesn't directly employ long-term care staff. Facilities are typically run by a municipality or not-for-profit."

There is a major issue with "valid "medical exemptions. Doctors are under the impression, based on claims by the government, that Covid-19 vaccines are safe in all groups. Therefore, women who are pregnant, lactating or planning to become pregnant, young children, those with autoimmune conditions or recovered from previous infection with Covid-19 do not qualify as a "valid" medical exemption. The exemption as stated just provides the government justification for claiming that they did not "force" anyone to receive the Covid-19 vaccine and that anyone who did receive the vaccine, did so willingly.

I attended a JET meeting this afternoon. Surprisingly, the PFAC was not on the agenda. After the meeting I sent an email to the members to remind them that I will not have internet access for seven days, beginning tomorrow.

October 10

I sent an email to the Seniors Online News to let them know that after November 1, I will no longer have access to inside health information. Therefore, I will not be able to provide the news updates as usual.

October 12

I chaired the PFAC meeting for the last time today. During the meeting, the two members complained about things that happened while I was away.

Potential PFAC members were vetted by JET Executive and the PFAC was not included. The existing selection process was not followed. There is PFAC agreement that the new members are good candidates, but the current members are displeased about not being included. This does not align with the Engagement Strategy.

PFAC will provide orientation to the new members.

We need to meet with the JET coordinator to discuss frustrations, to ensure that moving forward with new members, the process is followed, and engagement with JET is positive and meaningful.

We need to discuss current concerns now and remove them from the table, so they don’t bleed over to new members.

We need to present to the JET how the PFAC sees their role within the OHT and identify the mechanisms for us to be involved in the co-design.

Working groups have not reached out to PFAC for involvement. The group wonders why our input is not being sought. The engagement strategy states involvement from the beginning.

The government patient guideline incorporates the principle: "Nothing About Us Without Us."

The meeting frequency will be discussed once the new members have completed their orientation.

I committed to speak to the JET about the PFAC member

frustrations before I step down on November 1.

After the meeting, the secretary sent the above draft minutes to me for review and approval. I modified them to remove and negativity and returned the final minutes to the secretary for distribution to the JET and PFAC.

A few hours later, the secretary informed the PFAC that she had sent the draft minutes to the JET by mistake. I called the two members and said that the draft minutes did not mention that the comments came from them. The minutes made it look like I was the one doing the complaining. I told them that since I was stepping down on November 1, I will accept the blame. They need to remain neutral so that the PFAC will not fall apart.

October 14

I finalized the onboarding of the two new PFAC members and sent them an invitation for an Orientation meeting before the end of October.

Today provinces asked the Federal Government to consider the Johnson and Johnson single dose viral-vector Covid-19 vaccine, which was approved in February 2021, as an alternative to the mRNA vaccines. If the Feds agree, more people may be comfortable taking it.

October 15

I received an invitation to a Zoom meeting at 10:00 am with the PFAC Coordinator and the Hospital's Clinical Care manager.

I called the unvaccinated PFAC member and told her that I expect to be "fired" today. She told me that the two PFAC members were sent an invitation to a Zoom meeting at 11:00 am. We promised to call one another after our meetings.

During my call at 10:00 am, nothing was said about the minutes or the last PFAC meeting. The manager said that the JET were concerned about my mental health and thought that it was best for me to be relieved of my obligations immediately. The coordinator did not say anything. He just looked broken. My husband was in the other room and he heard everything. He was amazed that I did not lose my temper and that I even thanked them for their support.

After my meeting I called the PFAC member and said that my prediction was correct and that I had been fired, effective immediately. I encouraged her to suggest that the two remaining PFAC members co-Chair the committee. She thought that was the best way to advance the important work of the patient advisors.

After her meeting, she called me and said that they were both told that I would no longer chair the committee. They were not provided with a reason and were encouraged to remain as part of the team. She played her role and offered to co-chair and that suggestion was accepted.

I sent an email to my supervisor at the hospital and informed her that I would no longer be available to volunteer. I indicated that my workload and circumstances had changed.

Today is the day that I get my life back. No parents to care for and no volunteer work to occupy my days.

I spent the afternoon just reflecting on my volunteer work and purging my computer and email of OHT stuff. I still have my diary. It is unbelievable how many things I was involved in and the number of meeting minutes, documents and emails I generated over the past four years.

October 18

I prepared and recorded the news that I read in the media.

"The Simcoe Muskoka Health Unit reported 81new cases of Covid-19 for the past week. There were one 134 new cases reported the previous week. There were 5 deaths reported in September and one so far in October.

The Health Unit is concerned that Influenza will return with a vengeance this fall due to the reduction in restrictions that were in place last fall. Vaccination with Influenza vaccine is recommended for all ages.

All the preventative measures we took to fend off Covid-19 kept us clear of the influenza virus. But now that we're not keeping others at as much of a distance and we've let our guard down somewhat with widespread vaccination against Covid-19, there is expectation that not only will influenza return, but that it could hit hard.

The fear is that with little or no flu cases last year our immunity to it may not be as strong, meaning we may be more susceptible to it this year.

By early November, the general population will be able to access the flu vaccine at pharmacies and primary health-care facilities."

At this point, I had largely overcome the unexpected events of the previous Zoom meeting and proceeded to compose emails addressed to all members of JET, PFAC, and COHT with whom I had closely collaborated over the past four years. Everyone, except the coordinator, responded with positive messages. Interestingly, I did not hear from anyone that I did not send an email to, including the JET member who kept attacking me. It was my assumption that she was the reason I was fired and that the COHT had not been advised that I had been relieved of my duties earlier than expected. They would just assume that I decided not to be involved after November 1 and that is probably for the best.

October 21

A federal briefing said that the provinces and territories—who hold all the vaccination information—are responsible for providing the vaccine passport that Canadians need to travel internationally, using "existing provincial proof of vaccination systems". By 2022, all provinces and territories had "vaccine passports with the QR code that met the recommended Canadian standard for domestic and international travel".

The Ontario government announced a Covid-19 vaccine certification system that came into effect on September 22. It was met with protests.

October 25

I prepared and recorded the health news for the last time.

I felt such a sense of relief once I had completed this last volunteer task. I no longer need to put reminders in my calendar or schedule my life around meetings. I am now completely free to do what I want. Now, I just need to decide what it is that I want to do.

October 28

Some good news today. The Chief Medical Officer of Health of Ontario said that Ontario will not integrate a Covid-19 vaccine requirement into the Immunization of School Pupils Act (ISPA).

Chapter 22 – NOVEMBER 2021

November 3

I received an email today from the coordinator, who was forced to participate on the Zoom call that ended my 4-year volunteer career. He did not respond to my email in October, and I assumed that it took him a bit of time to get up the courage to contact me. For that matter, I heard that the PFAC members and many of the staff were instructed not to contact me. This is the message I received today.

"Hi Susan, thank you for your note and my apologies for the slow reply. You have been a true leader and have taken us through the most difficult of times (navigating Covid-19 and a completely new model of healthcare) over the last 3 years. I am proud to have had the pleasure of working closely with you and watching you as a PFAC chair and as a person. You bring passion to all that you do, and our PFAC has you to thank for its development and for providing a strong foundation for growth as our OHT continues to mature."

As I read this message, my self-esteem was restored and I promised myself to continue the fight against governments who lie and make promises they do not intend to keep.

November 19

The Public Health Agency of Canada announced upcoming adjustments to Canada's border measures. Included in the announced adjustments was the requirement for essential service providers, including truck drivers, to be fully vaccinated after January 15, 2022. The announcement clarified that unvaccinated or partially vaccinated foreign national truck drivers would be prohibited from entering Canada after that date. According to the Canadian Press and CBC, as of January 22, the mandates would impact an estimated 26,000 unvaccinated truckers of the 160,000 truck drivers in both the United States and Canada who regularly cross the border.

We headed into the second winter with Covid-19, and health agencies attempted to reach more vaccine-hesitant Canadians by making calls to those with a health card and who had not received any vaccine. This was one of the many concerns I expressed to the JET.

Chapter 23 – DECEMBER 2021

December 11

The number of daily Covid-19 cases were up to 1,600 – the highest number thus far. The number of vaccinated cases were 200 higher than the unvaccinated.

December 17

The Covid-19 case numbers were over 3,000 today with over 2,000 fully vaccinated.

December 23

The reported daily cases were up to 5,090, with over 4,000 in vaccinated individuals.

December 30

There were over 13,000 cases reported today. The number is probably an underestimation due to a shortage of Covid-19 tests. Most of the cases were in fully vaccinated.

Dr. Robert Malone joined Joe Rogan's podcast #1757 to discuss Covid-19 vaccines and related controversies. Malone discussed his background as an early developer of mRNA-vaccine technology and presented strong concerns about the safety, efficacy, and long-term effects of the Covid-19 mRNA vaccines. He argued that mass vaccination of low-risk groups, including children, was unnecessary and framed vaccine mandates as violation of informed consent and medical ethics.

When asked, Dr. Malone explained that after filing 19 patents for mRNA as a vaccine delivery system, he abandoned the research due to unresolved inflammation caused by the mRNA and non-localization of the product.

Dr. Malone described his infection with Covid-19 in February 2020, and the persistent Long-Covid symptoms he treated with re-purposed drugs. He was convinced by speaking with researchers that the issues he experienced with mRNA technology had been resolved by Moderna and that the vaccine may minimize his persistent symptoms, so he took the vaccine when the National Guard was offering it. When he received the vaccine, he was embarrassed to discover personally that those defects had not been eliminated and indeed the vaccine caused several severe adverse effects. Upon further investigation, he discovered that one of the ingredients used to make the lipid nanoparticles in the mRNA vaccines was polyethylene glycol (PEG). The nanoparticle was invented by the University of British Columbia and licensed to Moderna and Pfizer by UBC spin-off companies.

He was skeptical about the official treatment protocols, with heavy emphasis on hydroxychloroquine, ivermectin and drugs as potentially effective early-treatment options. He accused institutions of suppressing or distorting data on those drugs and the support of a one vaccine solution to the pandemic.

He and Rogan talked about content removal and de-platforming of vaccine-skeptic people, tying this to broader concerns about free speech and scientific debate.

The focus of the discussion was opposition to vaccine mandates, especially for children, with claims about under-reported risks such as myocarditis and possible long-term immune effects.

After the podcast was aired, there was considerable backlash and censorship. Malone was labelled as a mentally unstable conspiracy theorist, and Rogan was attacked for spreading dangerous misinformation.

Chapter 24 – JANUARY 2022

January 2

It was reported that over 18,000 cases were recorded today.

January 5

It was announced that restaurants, gyms and personal care will be closed for twenty-one days.

January 7

It was the first Friday of 2022. Something very alarming was happening. There were over 20,000 cases in one day and the majority of them were vaccinated. Closures, labour shortages, cancelled surgeries and diagnostics were not making any difference. We were heading into our third year of this pandemic. Side note - By June 22, 2022, the government stopped reporting Covid-19 cases by vaccination status.

January 15

It was reported that hydro chloroquine was being used to treat Multiple Sclerosis, Lupus and Rheumatoid Arthritis and was being tested in clinical trials for treatment of Covid-19. Based on this announcement and because the first three diseases were autoimmune disorders, I presumed that the severe effects of Covid-19 were also due to an autoimmune disorder induced by the virus.

January 17

Schools re-opened. Everyone was extremely nervous about sending their kids to school with the numbers increasing to unbelievable levels.

January 24

The Federal government ended exemptions for unvaccinated truckers crossing the US border, requiring them to quarantine upon return, despite about 90% of truckers already being vaccinated. This sparked outrage among the truckers and opponents of mandates.

In protest, a trucker in Alberta invited truckers to join him and his rig called Big Red heading for Ottawa. The stated goal of the Freedom Convoy began initially to oppose the federal government's Covid-19 vaccine mandate for cross-border truck drivers entering Canada. As the convoy reached Ottawa, the participants expanded their demands beyond trucker rules to call for an end to all federal Covid-19 restrictions and mandates.

January 28

The organizers of the Freedom Convoy stated that they just wanted an opportunity to speak to PM Trudeau about the unreasonable vaccine and mask mandates and would remain in Ottawa until that happened. They collected hundreds of trucks along the way and there was much support for them worldwide. Streets and bridges along their route were lined with Canadians cheering them on with Canadian flags.

Trudeau described the Freedom Convoy as a "fringe minority with unacceptable views". He also claimed that he must self-isolate due to contact with a person who tested positive for Covid-19. He went missing in action immediately after the announcement.

January 29

The Freedom Convoy was expected to arrive in Ottawa. There was also another trucker group headed to Ottawa who wanted Trudeau to step down and the government to dissolve. They arrived first and parked a large truck at the steps of the Parliament building with a huge sign cursing Trudeau and demanding his resignation.

Trudeau is still missing in action and there are different opinions and confusion on the news and social media about the two different groups of protesters.

January 30

The Freedom Convoy was expected to arrive today. They had decided to delay their arrival in Ottawa because Trudeau was still missing in action. Protests occurred in all capital cities across Canada today in support of the Freedom Convoy.

Two provinces, including Ontario, announced that they have

removed all mandates and will reopen tomorrow.

January 31

I was invited by Dr. Philip McMillan from Vejon Health to be a guest on his live programme to discuss the regulatory procedures for vaccines. I will join him on Saturday February 5. My husband and my son are concerned about the backlash but think that it is important for me to accept the invitation.

Chapter 25 – FEBRUARY 2022

February 5

The podcast with Dr. McMillan lasted one and a half hours with most of the time spent answering questions posed by him. The audience questions and comments began flowing in immediately and continued through the night.

One of the most difficult questions I was asked by Dr. McMillan was why other regulatory professionals were not willing to come forward and speak out about the vaccine regulatory process. It was a difficult question because I had no idea why individuals who trained in either the industrial or government regulatory field would allow obvious deviations from the process to be overlooked and withheld. Their tacit approval of the lies to the public will most probably tarnish the reputation of the profession and the vaccine industry for years to come.

February 6

I spent most of the day responding to questions on LinkedIn and YouTube.

A legal firm in Iowa contacted me to advise them on litigation against legislators. I turned them down.

February 7

I am still responding to comments resulting from the podcast. Many asked why I waited so long to express my concerns in public. My response was that I did attempt to raise concerns, however, I was censored by Facebook, Twitter and LinkedIn every time I tried. Now, I was grateful for the opportunity provided by Dr. McMillan to use his platform to get the message out.

February 12

The clash between the truckers and the Ottawa police is heating up.

February 14

To make the truckers leave Ottawa, Trudeau threatened to invoke the Emergency Act which is like Marshall Law. The invocation was supported by the Premier of Ontario. The rights and freedoms of Canadians would be further squashed if this was allowed to occur.

February 17

As part of the Emergency Act, bank accounts of convoy participants were locked, and three Freedom Convoy organizers were arrested. Side note - In late January 2024, a Canadian Federal court ruled that the government's use of the "Emergencies Act" to shut down the protest was unreasonable and had violated the Canadian Constitution.

February 19

I watched a great podcast with Dr. McMillan and Dr. Ross Jones, a retired pediatrician. They discussed whether the Covid-19 vaccines should be given to children. The main themes were that children were at low risk from Covid-19, the vaccines lacked long-term safety data, and the benefit-risk balance did not satisfy vaccinating healthy children.

The main concern was the novelty of the vaccine technology and the lack of long-term follow-up data. Dr. Ross focused on the low severity of Covid-19 in children and the ethical principle of avoiding harm to healthy patients. She also said that children should not be expected to bear vaccine risk for the sake of protecting older adults.

Surprisingly, I was mentioned twice in the podcast.

February 21

Dr. McMillan's podcast was deleted by LinkedIn along with several of my posts and we were both banned from the platform.

Coincidently, two books about vaccines that I ordered from Amazon were stopped at the border today. I received a message that they were returned to the sender.

These two incidents gave me a good indication of the censorship and tyranny existing in Canada and the US.

EPILOGUE

The Covid-19 pandemic had huge, overlapping impacts on health, economics, and social life, and is widely regarded as the most disruptive global crisis of the early 21st century.

It reshaped how people work, learn, and interact, and accelerated certain trends while exposing deep inequalities.

Disruptions to vaccination programs, maternal care, and chronic-disease management increased avoidable death rates.

Lockdowns, mask debates, and vaccine mandates increased social polarization, mistrust in institutions and misinformation.

By mid-August 2021, as Canada was facing a potential surge during the fourth wave of the highly contagious Delta variant, vaccinations were available to most adult Canadians, and many Canadians were vaccinated. As borders and schools were re-opening, so-called experts called for vaccine mandates.

In October 2021, the United States Department of Homeland Security (DHS) released new regulations regarding cross-border travel between Canada and the United States based on guidance from the Centers for Disease Control and Prevention (CDC). To prevent supply chain disruptions, the DHS allowed for a window of four months—until January 22, 2022—for Canadian truckers to get fully vaccinated against Covid-19.

Since October 29, 2021, proof of vaccination was mandatory for employees of federal public services and federally regulated industries, including banking. By early January, in these public sectors, those "without proof of vaccination, or a “valid” exemption on medical or religious grounds, were put on unpaid leave". Trudeau reinforced his comments about the unvaccinated people not allowed to board planes, trains and other federal transport. His comments ruled out alternatives like exemptions and testing.

In another interview, Trudeau stated that “Canadians know that the way to get through this pandemic is for everyone to get vaccinated. So, unless people have a “valid” medical exemption, they will not be able to board a plane or a train in Canada with vaccinated people.” He also announced that “By the end of October, if you’re 12 or older and want to fly or take a train, you’ll have to be fully vaccinated.”

Public reaction to Trudeau’s vaccine-based travel rules for planes and trains was sharply divided, with strong support from many Canadians who saw the rules as necessary for public health, and intense anger from others who viewed them as an overreach on personal freedom and questioned why testing for Covid-19 infection was not an acceptable alternative to vaccination.

The federal government was in dialogue along with other members of the Group of Seven nations, with the World Health Organization and the International Civil Aviation Organization to discuss international issues related to the global pandemic. This included proof of vaccination for international travel. As Canada was emerging from the fourth wave in mid-August 2021, in order to support the re-opening of societies and economies while also reducing the risk of spread and importation of Covid-19, the government concluded that Canadians needed to present proof of vaccination to Canadian and foreign border officials.

As a result, the ArriveCAN app was introduced for travellers arriving in Canada. The Canada Border Services Agency (CBSA) said that the ArriveCan app set the stage for a new system with technological changes to speed up entry to Canada at the border, starting with major airports. In order to be eligible for the exemption from quarantine and post-arrival testing requirements, travellers needed to submit their proof of vaccination which included the option of uploading it to ArriveCAN. By the summer of 2022, the app had become controversial, with border mayors calling for it to be scrapped.

In mid-April 2022 PM Trudeau made controversial comments linking unvaccinated individuals to racism and misogyny during a Quebec interview. He stated that a small group fiercely opposed to vaccination often consists of people who “don’t believe in science or progress and are very often misogynistic and racist,” questioning whether Canada should "tolerate these people". He and others labelled those who refused to receive the mRNA Covid-19 vaccine as anti-vaxxers. In fact, many of those who refused the shot were fully vaccinated with the routine vaccines and intended to continue.

In late April 2022, there were several news headlines that warned of vaccinated mixing with the "unvaccinated". The claim was that the unvaccinated were the cause of the large increases in the Covid-19 cases in vaccinated individuals and that the vaccinated were being infected by the unvaccinated. This claim was based on a fraudulent paper using a simulated computer model and commissioned by the Federal Government and published by the University of Toronto to support their vaccine mandates. The actual case reports categorised by vaccine status, did not corroborate the findings or assertions presented in the paper. In fact, the real data demonstrated the opposite effect. I wondered how the scientists could claim that uninfected, unvaccinated people who were forced to stay home could transmit the disease to vaccinated individuals. This was much more than lies by omission. This was a conspiracy to convince the masses that the unvaccinated among us were selfish and dangerous. It was another attempt by the government to create division among its voters.

The trend of vaccinated cases significantly outnumbering the unvaccinated continued until June 22, 2022, when the government curiously stopped reporting Covid-19 cases by vaccination status.

The fraudulent paper was neither withdrawn nor amended, despite several scientists and statisticians demanding a correction.

Another observation was the use of ventilators prior to the vaccine rollout. Any patient who was admitted to the ICU with severe Covid-19 was put on a ventilator, if it was available. Several of these patients died or sustained severe lung damage. Sometime in July 2022, the use of ventilators was significantly reduced, and patients were treated with anti-inflammatory drugs and high concentration oxygen. Fewer patients were dying under this treatment protocol. Not surprising, the vaccine was credited for the reduced death rate.

On February 23, 2023, Moderna announced a license agreement and hundreds of millions of dollars in payments to the US National Institutes of Health (NIH) for their key patent on the spike immunogen used in its Covid-19 vaccine. Dr. Fauci, who continued in his position of Director of the US National Institute of Allergy and Infectious Disease (NIAID), guided NIH funded work. He denied that the NIH was working at the Wuhan University on gain of function experiments with the Covid-19 virus. His denial was proven to be a lie. He assertively denied that Hydroxychloroquine or Ivermectin may be useful in treating Covid-19. The Lancet articles supporting his claims were later retracted after it was discovered that the data used to support the papers were fraudulent. Fauci should have announced a conflict of interest and stepped down from his advisory position during the pandemic.

In Canada, the University of British Columbia licensed their patent and received royalty payments in the millions of dollars via their spin-off companies from both Moderna and Pfizer for the use of their lipid nanoparticle delivery systems. This technology is essential for enabling mRNA vaccines to work effectively by delivering the mRNA to cells.

A point to keep in mind when following the money in the US and Canada is that under the Emergency Release regulations, if there are products on the market that could treat or prevent severe disease, no experimental products may be approved and released under the Emergency Release regulations. Therefore, if Ivermectin, Hydroxychloroquine, steroids and other products were made available off label for the treatment of severe Covid-19, the short-cuts taken with the mRNA vaccines would not be allowed and those companies and patent holders would not make the millions they made and are still making.

When the other products were used with success, the public was not made aware that there were treatments available to save lives. The vaccine continued to be credited for the drop in death rates.

In early 2023, Kevin McKernan first reported finding residual plasmid DNA (including bacterial plasmid-origin DNA and SV40-driven promoter/enhancer sequences) in mRNA- Covid-19-vaccine vials on the market. He described unexpected presence of these impurities in vials of both Pfizer and Moderna vaccines. He circulated a pre-print, which later became the subject of parliamentary and regulatory inquiries. The regulators would later confirm his findings, and his paper was published in September 2025.

SV40, which is a monkey virus, itself is classified as an oncogenic (cancer-causing) virus in animals. The regulators stated that they were not aware of the contaminants present in the vaccines when they were released for mass vaccination and assured the public that they now assessed the theoretical risks as very low. This is just another example of the short-cuts taken by the regulators when they allowed these experiential vaccines on the market.

The vaccines used in the early clinical trials that provided limited "safety and effectiveness data", were produced in small batches using a research manufacturing method. When the companies began scaling up their production to allow for mass immunization, vaccine batches produced by the scaled-up process were different than the batches produced for the clinical trials. Apparently, the regulators did not require retesting of the larger batches before they were mandated. This was a major oversight on the part of the regulatory profession.

On May 5, 2023, the WHO announced that Covid-19 no longer constituted a Public Health Emergency of International Concern.

They stated it remains a continuing long term health threat. This allowed the continued use of the vaccines under Emergency Release.

Many of those who received the Covid-19 vaccines and numerous booster shots suffered from severe adverse reactions, some resulting in death, or long-term health conditions. The rates of heart disease, vascular disease, cancer, autoimmune disease and dementia have increased many fold above the normal rates prior to the pandemic. The number of non- Covid-19 related deaths continue to climb in highly vaccinated countries.

In the spring of 2021, there were reports of myocarditis and pericarditis after mRNA Covid-19 vaccination, especially in younger males. On June 29, 2021, several Canadian published analyses using the Vaccine Adverse Event Reporting System data, quantified risks of using the mRNA vaccines. These reports built on the initial publication on May 28, 2021, that described 136 cases of myocarditis within 42 days' post-vaccination with a second dose, primarily in healthy males aged 16-30. In 2022, peer-reviewed publications described myocarditis as a recognized adverse event following mRNA vaccination. It was not until June 2025, that the FDA required updated prescribing information for mRNA Covid-19 vaccines to include warnings about myocarditis and pericarditis.

Although the risk was recognized in 2021, the regulators did not require formal label warnings until June 2025. Such a serious adverse event associated with a vaccine should have resulted in a product recall. Myocarditis is only one of the known serious adverse effects connected with the mRNA Covid-19 vaccines.

The numerous lockdowns, which did little to end the pandemic, produced large unintended harms across health, the economy and society. The debate is about how heavy-handed, prolonged and unevenly targeted they were compared with less disruptive alternative measures.

Mental health worsened sharply, with higher rates of anxiety, depression and stress-related conditions and many hospitals saw an increased use of mental-health services, and more emergency visits. Disruptions in non-covid care meant delayed diagnoses and treatment for cancer, heart disease and other serious conditions, sometimes leading to later stage, more serious conditions and death.

School closures were linked to learning loss, reduced cognitive and social-emotional development and increase in mental health issues.

Lockdowns caused widespread job losses, business closures and reduced economic growth. Higher poverty, housing instability and food-insecurity emerged.

It is a mystery to me, why they did not follow the Pandemic Influenza Plan developed in 2004 after the successful management of the SARS and H1N1 epidemics. The core goals of that plan are to prioritize saving lives through infection prevention, accelerated vaccine production (which they assumed would use the influenza production and formulation methods), and treatment access while navigating essential services. Lockdowns were considered more damaging than helpful and emergency release, vaccine mandates and coercion were not part of the plan.

Today in 2026, the world is still recovering from the negative impacts of the lockdowns, vaccine mandates, government overreach and loss of freedom of speech. It is difficult to foresee if the world will ever return to the pre-pandemic state.

During the pandemic, I was expelled from Twitter and LinkedIn for speaking the truth. I later discovered that the government ordered these platforms to close accounts of anyone who disagreed with their rhetoric.

When Elon Musk purchased Twitter, he promised to make it a forum for free speech. I rejoined in January 2023 and began posting more direct comments about the mandates, especially about the limited data for the mRNA vaccines at time of approval and the data now emerging about safety concerns and lack of effectiveness.

Although regulators and the public are aware of the safety concerns and lack of protection, the mRNA vaccines remain on the market. A recall would compromise the companies' ability to obtain approval for other vaccines using the same technology.

As predicted, there was an awakening taking place. Only a few Twitter readers disagreed with my posts and when they did disagree, they did so with abusive language and no data to support their position.

Life slowly returned to normal for me and my immediate family. Others went on to suffer long-term effects from the vaccine, long-covid or repeat Covid-19 infections. During the pandemic, I lost a mother due to neglect in an assisted living facility, one other family member due to complications after the vaccine, and two vaccinated family members from aggressive cancers. Recently, I heard from a member of our lunch group that she suffered and almost died from Guillian Barre just weeks after receiving a booster of the Covid-19 vaccine. I still hear stories about loved ones dying shortly after receiving the “shot”.

Young adults and their children who did receive the mRNA products, did so to either retain their job or their lifestyle. Many were coerced into taking something they were uncomfortable receiving.

Others who took the vaccine without any need for coercion, do not admit that they may have made the wrong decision. Those among us who are in denial will continue to support the actions taken by the government rather than admit to themselves that they were misled. I understand this attitude and can only hope that they at least admit it to themselves and do not fall for the lies again.

As predicted in 2021, several companies announced that the mRNA platform will be used to make all routine and future vaccines. Influenza was the first to be approved and released in 2025.

A societal shift has led to widespread vaccine distrust and the resurgence of preventable diseases, potentially causing more harm than the pandemic itself.

A significant issue arises should proof of the corruption among government officials, regulators, manufacturers and reporters come to light; such revelations could destabilize the entire health care system.

On a positive note, there were several important outcomes resulting from the pandemic.

Less reliance on the World Health Organization for pandemic management.

Several lessons learned about managing future pandemics.

The identification of risk factors for severe Covid-19 disease, Long-Covid and vaccine effects.

Treatments for acute Covid-19 and Long-Covid.

It was learned that ventilators should not be used when inflammation of the lungs is present. Reduction of inflammation using pharmaceutical products in combination with less invasive ventilation is the preferred protocol.

Improvements in hospital capacity and funding.

A review was initiated of vaccine schedules for children.

A re-evaluation of vaccine safety for children is planned.

New childhood vaccines will be not be approved by FDA without long-term safety studies.

Genetic testing for risk of serious adverse reaction to vaccines, including pediatric and Covid-19 vaccines is now possible.

There were several improvements in health care, home care, long-term care, retirement homes and mental health.

Ontario Health Teams were quickly advanced and funded in Ontario.

An awakening of society to government manipulation.

The creation of new social media platforms to enable free sharing of information without censorship.

The biggest disappointment to me during the Covid-19 vaccine roll-out and its continued use, was the failure of Regulatory professionals both in government and industry to do their jobs. Regulatory Affairs is a profession and corporate department that ensures organizations comply with local and global legislative guidelines. Regulatory professionals act as the crucial bridge between scientific innovation and government authorities to safeguard public health. Regulatory Affairs professionals are responsible for the entire lifecycle of a product.

Without Regulatory Affairs, safe and effective products would never successfully reach patients and consumers. This department translates raw laboratory and clinical data into the exact legal and scientific language that government regulators need to trust and approve a product for public use. Professionals in this area, constantly track evolving laws to protect the public from hazardous practices while ensuring companies can safely market their products.

It is my professional opinion that Regulatory executives working in companies who developed, manufactured and marketed the mRNA Covid-19 vaccines did not meet their professional obligations. I resigned Regulatory positions for much less than those "professionals" agreed to support.

When asked why more regulatory professionals were not speaking up, I allowed them the benefit of the doubt and was criticized for my defense of the profession. Today, I have no defense to offer.

Those of us who were lied to, mistreated, ignored, censored and slandered during the pandemic will and should never forget or forgive the atrocities carried out in the name of "science". We only need to follow the money and the transfer of power to understand who gained from the impact of the virus released from China.

Unfortunately, the world will continue to be ruled by those seeking financial gain and influence. It is up to us average citizens to keep them from repeating the perfect storm that was the Covid Pandemic.

If you have read the entire book, I thank you for your perseverance.

If you enjoyed this book, you may also be interested in my first book titled Sixth Sense – A Memoir.

Sixth Sense is the inspirational memoir of a young mother, who succeeded in a time and in an industry dominated by powerful men. When she was nineteen years old, she began her career as a junior laboratory technician at Connaught Medical Research Laboratories, a specialist in biologics, on the advice of her grandfather, a World War One Veteran. She struggled to balance family and career, while working her way through the ranks. After the birth of her son, she developed a debilitating condition, which was made worse by the demands of her job. By the age of forty, she had advanced to Vice President.

Her amazing journey takes us through the first two decades of her career and covers the AIDS and Ebola scares, the eradication of Smallpox, the Canadian Blood scandal, the Tylenol murders, and the evolution of biological therapeutics. It is set in a simpler time - a time of change, relative peace, social reform, yuppies, technological improvement, and a growing economy – a time of hope.

When asked to provide the reasons for her success the author said: “As the saying goes, behind every successful man is a good woman. In my case, there were two secrets behind my success - a good man and a sixth sense. I would not have had the strength to continue without my husband by my side. He was what kept me sane, what kept me balanced, and what allowed me to deal with the pressure. I was born with a sixth sense, which guided almost every decision I made, and frequently ensured that I was in the right place at the right time.”

www.ingramcontent.com/pod-product-compliance
Lightning Source LLC
Chambersburg PA
CBHW050521240926
51846CB00003B/647
9781972576397